OCCUPATIONAL THERAPY FOR ORTHOPAEDIC CONDITIONS

FORTHCOMING TITLES

Research Methods for Therapists
Avril Drummond

Group Work in Occupational Therapy
Linda Finlay

Stroke: Recovery and Rehabilitation
Polly Laidler

Caring for the Neurologically Damaged Adult
Ruth Nieuwenhuis

HIV and Aids Care
S. Singh and L. Cusack

Speech and Language Disorders in Children
Dilys A. Treharne

Spinal Cord Rehabilitation
Karen Whalley-Hammell

THERAPY IN PRACTICE SERIES

Edited by Jo Campling

This series of books is aimed at 'therapists' concerned with rehabilitation in a very broad sense. The intended audience particularly includes occupational therapists, physiotherapists and speech therapists, but many titles will also be of interest to nurses, psychologists, medical staff, social workers, teachers or volunteer workers. Some volumes are interdisciplinary, others are aimed at one particular profession. All titles will be comprehensive but concise, and practical but with due reference to relevant theory and evidence. They are not research monographs but focus on professional practice, and will be of value to both students and qualified personnel.

Occupational Therapy for Orthopaedic Conditions

DINA PENROSE

Head Occupational Therapist, Royal Orthopaedic Hospital,
Birmingham, UK

CHAPMAN & HALL
London · Glasgow · New York · Tokyo · Melbourne · Madras

Published by Chapman & Hall, 2-6 Boundary Row, London SE1 8HN

Chapman & Hall, 2-6 Boundary Row, London SE1 8HN, UK

Blackie Academic & Professional, Wester Cleddens Road, Bishopbriggs, Glasgow G64 2NZ, UK

Chapman & Hall, 29 West 35th Street, New York NY10001, USA

Chapman & Hall Japan, Thomson Publishing Japan, Hirakawacho Nemoto Building, 6F, 1-7-11 Hirakawa-cho, Chiyoda-ku, Tokyo 102, Japan

Chapman & Hall Australia, Thomas Nelson Australia, 102 Dodds Street, South Melbourne, Victoria 3205, Australia

Chapman & Hall India, R. Seshadri, 32 Second Main Road, CIT East, Madras 600 035, India

Distributed in the USA and Canada by Singular Publishing Group Inc., 4284 41st Street, San Diego, California 92105

First edition 1993

© 1993 Dina Penrose

Typeset in 10/12 point Times Roman by DSC Corporation Ltd., Cornwall, England

Printed in Great Britain by St Edmundsbury Press, Bury St Edmunds, Suffolk

ISBN 0 412 39370 0   1 56593 044 4 (USA)

 Printed on permanent acid-free text paper, manufactured in accordance with the proposed ANSI/NISO Z 39.48-199X and ANSI Z 39.48-1984

Contents

Acknowledgements

I am indebted to many staff of all disciplines at the Royal Orthopaedic Hospital, Birmingham, for their help so willingly given during the preparation of this book.

I wish to acknowledge the help given by medical staff in their particular areas of interest: Mr C. Bradish (limb length discrepancy), Mr Simon Carter (bone tumours), Dr P. Grigoris (hip and knee replacements and revision surgery) and Mr M. Waldram (hand surgery). I also with to thank Mr J.C.T. Fairbank (Nuffield Orthopaedic Centre, Oxford, formerly of the Royal Orthopaedic Hospital) for his help with the section on low back pain and spinal surgery.

I am grateful to Lynda Gwilliam, occupational therapist at the Hand Unit, Wrightington Hospital, Wigan, for her help with rehabilitation following surgery to the hand and elbow in rheumatoid arthritis, and to Tina Dolan, occupational therapist at the Disablement Services Centre, Selly Oak, for her assistance over wheelchairs and artificial limbs. My thanks to Frances Burton, occupational therapist with Wiltshire Social Services (formerly of the Royal Orthopaedic Hospital) and to Jan Puddephatt, tutor at the West Midlands School of Occupational Therapy, for reading my first draft, and for their helpful suggestions and comments.

Thanks are also due to Judy Dawson, Librarian at the Research and Teaching Centre, Royal Orthopaedic Hospital, for obtaining reference works; the Medical Illustration Department, Selly Oak Hospital, for printing the X-ray photographs; Mr R. Grimer (Consultant, Bone Tumour Service) for permission to use the illustrations of bone tumour surgery; Josie Cardall for her help with the preliminary typing and for being my general factotum throughout; and to Ann Weaver for putting the manuscript on to a word processor.

Lastly I must record my gratitude to my husband Patrick, for his patience and support, and for keeping me 'fed and watered' as I worked.

Dina Penrose
Birmingham

Preface

This book is written with occupational therapy students in mind, as a guide to newly qualified occupational therapists and for those returning to work after a break in service. Over the years I have been asked many times by newly appointed staff whether I could recommend a book to prepare them for working with orthopaedic patients. I hope this small volume will fill the gap in the literature on the subject, and that it will be useful as a quick reference book. I hope it may also fall into the hands of those in other disciplines and enable them to understand and appreciate the contribution of the occupational therapist to the rehabilitation team.

This is the era of joint replacement, with ever-increasing demand for primary and revision surgery. Improved implants and improved surgical techniques are constantly being researched. Surgery for bone tumour is less mutilating and more hopeful than ever before. Operations to release tendons and soft tissue contractures, tendon transfers, osteotomies, spinal fusion, joint fusion, etc. are performed on patients with neurological problems, thus improving function and appearance and preventing further deformity. These are some examples of procedures in this exciting and fast-developing field, while hospital beds are occupied for an ever shorter period of time and the potential for occupational therapy is enormous. 'If surgery is to be successful, the importance of assessing the patient as a human being cannot be over-emphasised' (Souter, 1987). This is precisely the approach of the occupational therapist.

The reader is expected to be familiar with the anatomy and physiology of the locomotor system. Background information on the conditions presenting for elective orthopaedic surgery (i.e. operations planned in advance) is included, to enable the reader to understand the processes which are taking place within the patient's body and mind. Results of surgery are also presented to give an informed overall picture.

While orthopaedics and trauma tend to be mentioned in tandem, it is not within the scope of this book to include trauma, which is a vast subject in its own right, requiring a companion volume.

For convenience I have used the personal pronoun 'he' when referring to the patient or surgeon, and 'she' when referring to the physiotherapist or occupational therapist.

In an attempt to avoid monotonous repetition, I have used synonyms such as joint replacement and arthroplasty, indwelling prosthesis and implant, and elective and cold orthopaedic surgery.

REFERENCE

Souter, W.A. (1987) Surgical management of rheumatoid arthritis, in S.P.F. Hughes, M.K. Benson and C. Colton (eds.) *Orthopaedics: The principles and practice of musculoskeletal surgery*, Churchill Livingstone, Edinburgh.

1

Rheumatoid arthritis

Rheumatoid arthritis is a chronic, inflammatory, systemic disease, affecting multiple joints and characterized by periods of exacerbation and remission. The small joints are usually affected first, and joint involvement is usually symmetrical.

THE DISEASE PROCESS

The synovial membrane is hypertrophied, highly vascular and packed with inflammatory cells. This aggressive tissue:

- erodes cartilage and subchondral bone;
- infiltrates tendon mechanisms, restricting glide, and can ultimately lead to tendon rupture;
- invades connective tissue;
- produces sensory and motor nerve compressions, especially in closed compartments such as the median nerve as it passes beneath the flexor retinaculum in the carpal tunnel.

The results of this tissue invasion are:

- pain
- instability
- contracture
- muscle weakness
- subluxation and deformity.

The degree of damage and the individual's perception of the disease will result in varying degrees of functional loss.

Phases of the disease

The disease can be arbitrarily divided into three phases: acute, sub-acute and chronic.

The acute phase is characterized by inflamed, swollen, painful joints, general malaise and raised temperature.

During the sub-acute phase the disease is less active and better controlled by medication. The patient's condition remains stable for longer periods of time, but joint deformity is progressing.

By the chronic phase the disease is no longer active, but the residual mechanical problems in and around the joints will produce pain, instability or stiffness, resulting in loss of function.

Management of the disease

Management of the disease is largely medical, but therapeutic measures and surgical intervention can minimize the effects of the disease. Evaluations and treatment are an ongoing process, and the multidisciplinary team approach, involving rheumatologist, orthopaedic surgeon, nurses, physiotherapist, occupational therapist, orthotist and social worker, is essential.

During the acute phase medical management frequently involves admission to hospital for complete or partial bedrest. During the sub-acute phase, limitation of physical activity will be in keeping with the systemic and local manifestations of the disease. A vast selection of drugs are also used to control rheumatoid arthritis. They include:

- analgesics
- non-steroid anti-inflammatory drugs (NSAIDs)
- corticosteroids
- intramuscular gold injections
- injections of hydrocortisone directly into the joint.

Careful monitoring of the effects of these drugs on the patient is essential, as many have unpleasant and potentially dangerous side effects. The hydrocortisone injections give long-lasting relief, but repeated injections cause destruction of the cartilage. Anaemia is common in the acute phase, due to the sequestering of iron in the tissues, but as this resolves on remission iron supplements are unnecessary.

SURGICAL INTERVENTION

This must be preceded by careful evaluation of the patient and their problems. This is often carried out by the occupational therapist in consultation with the surgeon, rheumatologist and physiotherapist. The process of deformity in the rheumatoid limb is complex, and no single procedure can give the desired result. The combination of operations must be chosen which will give the patient the best possible pain relief and restoration of function with the least number of hospital admissions. The patient's total physical condition must also be considered, e.g. it would be very unwise to perform bilateral wrist replacements on a patient who has gross lower limb problems, as the punishment imposed on the wrists by the use of crutches would lead to early deterioration of the implants. It is much wiser to defer hand surgery until the lower limbs have received attention. If this is not possible it would be preferable to settle for one wrist arthrodesis for strength, and one arthroplasty for dexterity.

When deciding the course of action, the patient's attitudes, expectations and ability to cope must be taken into account. Clear explanations, including the advantages and limitations of surgery, must be given, and specific goals must be set against which to measure post-operative results.

The general rule for upper limb surgery is to work from proximal to distal, as a hand that cannot be positioned adequately, or have power transmitted through it because of pain or instability at proximal joints, is reduced in function. In addition to the proximal to distal rule, certain priorities should be observed, in particular that nerve compressions should be dealt with as a matter of urgency, and tendon compressions should be a very close second. Because of her close and frequent contact with the patient, the occupational therapist is often the first to notice these compressions, and the need for vigilance cannot be over-emphasized.

The aims of surgery are to:

1. relieve pain;
2. maintain and improve function;
3. prevent further deterioration;
4. improve appearance.

The patient should be in a sub-acute or chronic phase of the disease before surgery is performed. Surgery may be preventive, or of a repair or reconstructive nature. An example of the former is synovectomy, which is performed to prevent the bulky hypertrophic synovium further damaging a joint. Examples of repair or reconstructive surgery are repair of ruptured extensor tendons of the fingers, and osteotomy to re-align a defective limb. While joint replacements will be the main surgery under discussion, it must be stated that arthrodesis, principally of the wrist, thumb and PIP joints, is a viable surgical option. The aim is to achieve a balance between optimum function or mobility and optimum stability.

As orthopaedic surgery has made dramatic advances in recent years, the range of procedures available for the rheumatoid upper limb has expanded accordingly. From simple excision arthroplasty has evolved the use of implant surgery, with implants available for shoulder, elbow, ulnar head, wrist, MCP and PIP joints of the fingers and the thumb. The various surgical procedures will be discussed in the relevant chapters.

To summarize surgery for the rheumatoid upper limb:

1. Meticulous surgery is essential as the tissues are delicate and the deformities complex.

2. It is important to recognize that the disease still exists, although the joints may have been replaced, and that therapeutic and prophylactic measures are still appropriate.
3. It is not uncommon for patients to go through a phase of 'flare-up' following surgery, and appropriate systemic and local measures must be employed.
4. Realistic goals must be set, as a complete return to normal is not possible.
5. Treatment must be a co-ordinated effort between the members of the multidisciplinary team.

A brief mention must be made of certain surgical procedures which are frequently encountered on the orthopaedic ward, and which are employed in the surgical management of rheumatoid arthritis. One is ankle arthrodesis, either fusion of the talo-tibial joint, or a triple arthrodesis of the talo-calcaneo, talo-navicular and calcaneo-cuboid joints, both of which offer good pain relief. Ankle replacement has become available, and would benefit the rheumatoid patient as in theory it would be preferable to the impact forces transmitted upwards to other joints after arthrodesis. However, considerable muscle power would be required to stabilize such a joint (Souter, 1987).

The spine is affected most noticeably in the cervical area. At the atlanto-axial joint, erosion of the odontoid process produces an unstable joint with subluxation, endangering the spinal cord. A rigid collar worn day and night is supplied as a matter of urgency, and fusion of the cervical spine may be indicated, after which a closely moulded collar is fitted before the patient is allowed to mobilize.

THERAPEUTIC MANAGEMENT

The occupational therapist and physiotherapist, working together, can complement each other's treatments and reinforce each other's teaching. The occupational therapist, as part of the multidisciplinary team, can make a considerable contribution to the patient's well-being by helping to relieve pain, improving functional ability and aiding psychological adjustment to disability.

Depending on the clinical phase of the disease, the objectives of treatment are:

1. to educate and reassure the patient about the disease;
2. to instruct in the methods of energy conservation, and explain the benefits;
3. maintain or increase joint mobility;
4. maintain or increase strength and endurance;
5. prevent or minimize, by appropriate splinting, adaptations and joint protection techniques, the effects of the disease on the joint structures;
6. maintain or improve function, enabling the patient to achieve maximum independence;

7. provide the environment, support and advice to facilitate the individual's psychological adjustment to disability;
8. resettle the patient at home, work and socially.

Splinting

Splinting is frequently used during all phases of the disease. Its use may be therapeutic, prophylactic, functional, pre-operative or post-operative.

Therapeutic splinting decreases joint pressure and inflammation by eliminating painful movement and reflex muscle spasm during the acute phase of the disease. An example of this type of splinting is the resting splint for the hand and wrist. This splint supports the joint structures and discourages muscle spasm, which increases pain and encourages positions of deformity, notably at the metacarpophalangeal (MCP) and proximal interphalangeal (PIP) joints. The resting splint positions the wrist in slight ulnar deviation and maximum painfree extension up to 30°, the thumb in abduction and opposition, the MCP joints in zero deviation and functional flexion of 30°, and the PIP joints in 10–15° of flexion. The wearing of the resting splint during the acute phase is balanced with gentle passive or active exercise to the point of discomfort, without stretching, at least twice daily.

Prophylactic splinting is used both during and immediately following an acute phase, and during the sub-acute phase. Prophylactic splinting aims to maintain optimum joint alignment for function, and to prevent contractures developing in non-functional positions. Although there is no concrete evidence that prophylactic splinting prevents joint deformities by minimizing dynamic forces, there is enough clinical evidence to make it worthwhile. An example of such a splint is the MCP joint stabilizer, which aims to prevent ulnar deviation at the MCP joints.

Functional splinting is aimed at unstable or painful joints and is used extensively during the sub-acute and chronic phases of the disease. Painful, unstable joints cannot transmit power, therefore function is impaired. This is particularly true of the wrist joint, where pain and instability inhibit finger flexor power. A wrist support will stabilize the joint and eliminate pain on movement, and frequently results in dramatically improved hand function.

Pre-operative splinting is used to stretch soft tissue contractures to facilitate surgery.

Post-operative splinting is used extensively following reconstructive surgery to the upper limb. It aims to:

1. provide mobility in prescribed arcs of movement;
2. assist in post-operative strengthening;
3. prevent or minimize post-surgical adhesions;

4.   maintain surgically achieved alignment.

Examples of these splints will be described with the relevant surgery.

OCCUPATIONAL THERAPY ASSESSMENT

By the time the patient with rheumatoid arthritis needs surgery, there will be considerable joint damage and probably deformity.

A complete occupational therapy assessment covers local environmental aspects and function, including the social and psychological needs of the patient. Observation shows that by this stage many patients will have ceased to be in employment. Housewives are usually working in that they are performing household tasks.

At their first meeting the therapist may gently shake hands with the patient. This can give considerable information to the therapist in an informal way, at least so far as the right hand is concerned! Power, deformity, subluxation, skin temperature and sweating can be roughly estimated. This introduction gives the therapist the opportunity to explain her role to the patient.

If joint measurement has been carried out by the physiotherapist it is pointless to duplicate the exercise. As the patient's condition fluctuates frequently and varies according to the time of day, the assessment is better carried out over several sessions. This is less tiring for the patient and enables a repetition of some tests, if this is thought desirable.

Pressures of time often lead to therapists utilizing a checklist of questions as to whether patients are able to perform activities, but results are often inaccurate. Compared to answering a therapist's questions at a personal interview, patients appear to admit to difficulties more readily in a self-administered questionnaire (Speigel *et al.*, 1985). It is preferable for the occupational therapist to take the patient through a practical assessment.

The activities of daily living (ADL) assessment must include:

1.   personal care: dressing, washing and bathing, toileting and hygiene, grooming and feeding;
2.   mobility: walking, stair management, transfers on and off chair, bed and possibly wheelchair;
3.   housework: cooking, cleaning, laundry, shopping, handling money;
4.   supporting activities: lifting, reaching for, handling and carrying objects;
5.   communication: writing, use of telephone, handling a book.

Various assessment forms have been devised for the recording of ADL assessment. One form covering assessment of the above activities under broad headings (Figure 1.1) and a second form breaking down dressing activities, including putting on and removing splints and other appliances (Figure 1.2), should suffice. Grading makes for concise reporting.

South Birmingham Health Authority

OCCUPATIONAL THERAPY

ASSESSMENT REPORT

NAME: REG NO.

ADDRESS   AGE:

ACTIVITY	DATE
CHAIR MANAGEMENT	
WALKING	
CLIMB STAIRS	
IN AND OUT OF BED	
DRESS	
MANAGE OWN TOILET	
WASH	
SHAVE	
COMB HAIR	
IN AND OUT OF BATH	
ABLE TO FEED	
MAKE POT OF TEA	
MAKE LIGHT MEAL	
COOK DINNER	
TIDY BED	
LIGHT CLEANING	

REMARKS   SIGNED

                                    OCCUPATIONAL THERAPIST

Figure 1.1 Sample form for general ADL assessment

ROYAL ORTHOPAEDIC HOSPITAL - BIRMINGHAM, 31

OCCUPATIONAL THERAPY DEPARTMENT

NAME: NUMBER:

ADDRESS: DATE OF BIRTH:

ACTIVITY	DATE	DATE	DATE	DATE
GARMENTS OVER HEAD				
SHIRT/CARDIGAN/COAT				
PANTS/TROUSERS				
SOCKS/STOCKINGS/TIGHTS				
SHOES				
SMALL BUTTONS				
ZIPS				
SHOELACES				
TIE				
APPLIANCE/CALIPER				
HAT				
GLOVES				

KEY TO GRADING   1) Independent, using aids if necessary

                            2) Needs to be talked through activity

                            3) Minimal assistance needed

                            4) Considerable assistance needed

                            5) Unable to perform activity

REMARKS: SIGNED:

                    OCCUPATIONAL THERAPIST

Figure 1.2 Sample form for dressing assessment

This form should also record what aids were used, how long the activity took to complete, how tired the patient became and what action is necessary to improve performance.

If a patient does well in his ADL assessment, it must be remembered that while he can cope in the hospital setting, he may not manage so well on discharge, when he has to contend with every task, both personal and domestic, on a daily basis.

Hand assessment may be required. This is covered in Chapter 9.

For many patients a pre-discharge home assessment is necessary. During this the occupational therapist assesses:

1. the patient's ability to get in and out of a car, and instruct accordingly;
2. mobility outdoors from car to front door, and indoors over carpets and on stairs;
3. accessibility and layout of the home: steps, stairs, doorways, etc.;
4. position of toilet and bathroom in relation to living room, bedroom and stairs;
5. arrangement of furniture in relation to access and mobility;
6. accessibility of electric power points;
7. accessibility of regularly used utensils and foodstuff;
8. hazardous loose mats and other obstacles: these must be identified and their removal negotiated;
9. availability of adequate, nourishing food supply in the pantry;
10. patient's ability to get in and out of an armchair, on and off bed and toilet, in and out of bath or shower, if appropriate;
11. patient's ability to make hot drink;
12. patient's ability to operate heating system;
13. whether the light switch is operable from the bed;
14. whether the patient can summon help if he lives alone.

Aids in situ should be noted, those needed should be noted and requisitioned, and inappropriate equipment should be removed and replaced if necessary with more suitable models.

If a work assessment is required, the therapist should enquire as to what the patient's job involves, the working conditions, and how he travels there. Details of work assessment are covered in Chapter 12.

Because of the far-reaching effects of rheumatoid arthritis in terms of pain, disability and deformity, there are profound psychological effects on the patient. In her assessment the therapist should include her estimate of the patient's attitude towards his disease, disability and appearance, and whether he is resentful, angry, frustrated or depressed.

An education programme in a group setting, giving accurate information about the disease, suitable literature, benefits available, diet, tools and adaptations for daily living, is helpful. It is important that both patient and family members are correctly informed, otherwise they may obtain inaccurate information from a lay source.

JOINT PROTECTION PROGRAMME

Since trauma aggravates an arthritic joint, the concept of joint protection arose. The aims of joint protection are to relieve pain and to help prevent deformity and further damage to joints. The principles of joint protection are to:

1. use proper body mechanics, i.e. use the strongest joint to perform a task, e.g. use hips and knees for lifting rather than the spine, push rather than pull heavy objects, slide objects along the ground and along worktops, and use wheels where possible rather than lift or carry;
2. use each joint in its most stable plane, e.g. approach activities squarely, such as standing directly in front of a drawer to open it;
3. spread the load of lifting or carrying over several joints, e.g. carry a tray across the forearms;
4. maintain range of movement and muscle strength, e.g. fully flex and extend the elbows when sweeping or ironing;
5. avoid activities which encourage ulnar drift, e.g. use of small handles or wringing out cloths;
6. avoid prolonged static grasp of tools, etc., e.g. knitting, crochet, holding a book to read it;
7. avoid overdoing an activity, respect pain when it occurs, and stop to rest;
8. wear any splints provided.

The patient should be taught to recognize and avoid activities which:

1. put pressure on the radial side of any finger;
2. put strong pressure on the thumb.

As alternative hobbies to knitting or crochet, bilateral hand activities such as weaving and macrame should be suggested. A remedial exercise for ulnar drift is to place the hand flat on the table, then move each finger in turn up and over towards the thumb.

Positioning of the joints at rest is part of the joint protection programme. Because of generalized pain, patients are apt to rest with pillows under the knees. This should be discouraged, as it may lead to the development of flexion contractures of the hips and knees. At rest the legs should be straight, with the feet supported at right angles to prevent the development of equinus deformity. If there is a tendency to flexion deformity at hips or knees, some part of each day should be spent lying prone on a single bed. The feet must be over the edge of the bed to prevent equinus deformity.

Joints may be protected from deformity if a joint protection programme is implemented soon after diagnosis. When damage has already occurred the application of the principles will still be beneficial in delaying further deterioration and relieving pain.

ENERGY CONSERVATION

In the early stages of the disease a patient may try to maintain former activity levels, and push himself too hard. Energy conservation is, therefore, important at this stage and for patients in whom the disease process is more advanced. The concept is closely allied to joint protection. To conserve energy the patient should:

1. have at least one daily rest of an hour or more;
2. balance rest and activity, e.g. by working for 20 minutes, then resting for five minutes, etc.;
3. pace work, so that only a little heavy work is done daily, interspersed with light tasks;
4. use labour-saving equipment where possible;
5. arrange equipment and materials within easy reach;
6. adjust work surfaces to a suitable height for the job in hand;
7. sit rather than stand;
8. learn to accept help when it is necessary;
9. learn to eliminate unnecessary tasks.

Tools for living are provided as enabling devices and to protect the joints from damage by avoiding positions which cause deformity. While the occupational therapist will discuss the foregoing with the patient, and explain the how and why of joint protection and energy conservation, there is a limit to how much the patient can retain, so many Occupational Therapy departments give patients booklets setting down this information and giving details of suitable tools for living. The booklets are written for easy understanding and suggest various methods for putting the principles into practice and sources of supply for the tools. If it is of A5 size, the patient is more likely to keep it on his bookshelf.

The United States Department of Health and Human Services published a workbook in 1985 entitled *Rehabilitation Through Learning* (Furst *et al.*, 1985). Its aim was to enable people wishing to take some responsibility for managing their illness to do so with help from professionals and their own family. The workbook comprised four units as follows:

1. **Body position**: patients to note daily what energy-draining positions they observe, the cause and solution.

2. **Rest**: patients time activities, noting rest periods, and record the scale of pain and fatigue following the activity. This enables the planning of more appropriate rest periods.

3. **Activity analysis**: patients break down a selected activity into component parts, decide on rest breaks, consider body position, work surface heights, location of materials and what gadgets will be used. Also make a weekly timetable, spreading out heavy tasks. At the end of each day the tasks completed are ticked and any remaining are redistributed.

4. **Joint protection**: worksheets help patients distinguish 'normal' joint pain from that caused by overdoing activities. Pain should wear off within an hour of finishing an activity. Other worksheets record whether patients use joint protection methods of which they are aware.

In 1987 a research paper published in the *American Journal of Occupational Therapy* compared the results of traditional energy conservation training with the results achieved after using this workbook-based programme for three months. Follow-up of patients having had traditional training suggested that the methods were not effective in changing patients' behaviour. Conversely, using the workbook-based programme, 67% of patients had improved in measures of pain and fatigue and 47% were more physically active. This suggests that the development of behavioural awareness and problem-solving skills gave the patients some measure of control over their disease (Furst *et al.*, 1987).

COUNSELLING

When a person is first told he has rheumatoid arthritis he is shocked and becomes anxious and possibly depressed. He has, in fact, to go through the stages of grieving for his lost health. By the time he needs orthopaedic surgery he has recovered from the initial shock, but is still subject to bouts of depression. This is a normal response to having to adapt to live with a painful, potentially disfiguring disease. Occasionally antidepressant drug therapy may be required if the depression syndrome is present: i.e. disturbed sleep, weight loss, apathy, etc.

The patient may be pre-occupied with his symptoms, and needs help in expressing his fears. If he feels he has lost control over his life, he is likely to be angry, but he cannot easily express this openly because he needs the help of his family and the hospital staff and feels he cannot take it out on them.

The body image of the patient with rheumatoid arthritis may take a hard knock. He may have to suffer the indignity of difficult mobility and possible visible deformity, and if on steroids, his appearance is further altered by the development of a fat 'moon' face.

In an informal setting the patient can be encouraged to verbalize his fears, anger and resentment, and must be reassured that these feelings are normal. He must be treated with respect, recognizing that he has sentiments and aspirations like anybody else, and this will have a positive effect on his self-esteem. Careful listening to the patient is helpful, just to let him express his frustration. It will also demonstrate if he has any misconceptions about the disease and enable these to be rectified. The patient's problems should not be minimized, but he should know that although prognosis is difficult, most patients do not develop severe disability and that, by following the joint protection and energy conservation programmes, he can take some control over his disease.

The patient's partner or family may also need counselling. Their attitudes depend on their relationship before the onset of the illness. They may be overprotective, resentful, etc. They may find commitment to a long period of care daunting, and their plans for the future are in limbo. Some partners respond positively and selflessly, while others cannot cope with the situation and withdraw from it, with the possibility of divorce. Frequently there is role reversal, especially where the breadwinner becomes arthritic, and this may be hard for both partners to accept, leading to the loss of self-esteem on the one hand and possible resentment on the other. Any financial loss imposes further strain. The social worker's help may be invaluable here. The carer must be advised against becoming so wrapped up in the patient's care that he becomes socially isolated, and he will do his caring job better if he takes time off for recreation.

If the patient needs help with intimate functions such as bathing or toileting, this is degrading. Such problems should be discussed with the occupational therapist, who is best placed to resolve the difficulty and promote maximum independence and dignity in the patient.

PROMOTION OF INDEPENDENCE

Mobility

The occupational therapist supplements the physiotherapist's treatment for mobility. Many patients eventually need a walking aid, and a walking stick is often sufficient. It is important that it is of the correct height: if too short the patient will stoop, if too long the wrist is forcibly extended, thus damaging the joint. To obtain the correct length, the patient should be wearing his normal shoes, stand erect, and be measured from the greater trochanter to the ground. Alternatively, the stick should be placed upside down on the ground and the length marked on the stick at the wrist crease. Any surplus is sawn off, and the ferrule re-applied. The ferrule should be wide-based and regularly renewed. The stick should be held in the hand opposite the affected leg, so that the body weight is transferred through the arm and thence through the stick. If two sticks are needed the patient is taught the four point gait pattern, i.e. one stick forward, then the opposite foot, second stick forward, then the second foot.

If crutches are needed, the physiotherapist will assess for them and teach their use, but the occupational therapist must monitor their correct use when carrying out her part of the rehabilitation programme. Axillary crutches are contra-indicated, because of the danger of damage to the gleno-humeral joint. Forearm crutches are more weight-relieving than sticks. The length of the crutches should be adjusted so that the elbows are held in 15–20° of flexion. The handles of sticks and crutches may need padding or moulding for the individual patient. Fischer sticks are useful for this reason. If thumbs are severely affected, gutter crutches may be necessary, well padded along the gutter. The height should be adjusted so that the shoulders are not hunched, and the same applies to pulpit frames. For all walking aids, wide-based ferrules are essential.

A wheelchair may be needed for outdoor use, to enable carers to take the patient out shopping or socially. Thought must be given as to whether the patient is to propel the wheelchair himself or whether it is to be attendant pushed, the latter being more likely. If severely disabled, even if temporarily so, assessment for elevating legrests, extended backrest, etc. may be needed. Cushioning to protect the ischial tuberosity area is necessary and anti-pressure cushioning may be indicated. The depth of the cushioning affects the balance of the patient in the wheelchair. A powered wheelchair or scooter may enable the individual to achieve greater independence out of doors.

If a wheelchair is needed for indoor use, an electrically powered model should be considered at an early stage, as it helps to preserve function in the upper limbs and conserves energy. The home must be assessed to ensure that there is enough space to get through doors, to turn around and to determine whether ramps are needed. A patient who cannot stand to transfer needs a model with removable arms plus a transfer board, and patient and carer must be trained in their use.

Seating

Correct seating is essential. If the patient's armchair is unsuitable his pain is aggravated and his independence adversely affected in that he finds it difficult to get up to go to the toilet, get his meals, answer the door, etc.

It is surprising how few patients with rheumatoid arthritis have suitable chairs. This may be due to cost, or perhaps they have left it too long before obtaining one, so that going out to buy one has become virtually impossible. The nearest Disabled Living Centre will supply details of furniture dealers and manufacturers who will visit a patient at home to try out chairs. Social Services departments may supply a chair, but many provide only the means of raising them, which may be inadequate for the rheumatoid patient. If Social Services state that they cannot supply a chair, the social worker can approach a charity, such as Arthritis Care, for help with funding.

The Disabled Living Centre is the best place to go for assessment for a suitable armchair. They usually have a good range of chairs and the patient receives the undivided attention of the therapist. It is important to allow plenty of time and when a chair seems right, the patient should sit in it for 20–30 minutes, because sometimes a chair feels right at first but becomes intolerable after ten minutes or so.

When assessing for an armchair, the following points should be considered:

- The patient should wear his usual house shoes.
- Choose firm fabric upholstery (vinyl causes sweating).
- Seat height should be from floor to the bend behind the knees, with knees at right angles and feet resting flat on the floor.
- Seat depth is from back of buttocks to bend behind the knees, minus one to two inches (2.5 to 5-cm).
- Seat width should be the width at the hips plus four inches (10cm) each side to allow for changing position.
- Backrest contours should support the whole length of the spine, including the head.
- Backrest angle to suit the individual.
- Armrests should support the arms, without hunching the shoulders.
- Armrests should be level or sloping upwards at the front, reaching right to the front of the chair to assist in rising. A shaped wooden handgrip is helpful.
- Armrests should be padded to accommodate painful elbows and rheumatoid nodules.
- No crossbar to brace front legs of chair, as this impedes rising.

More severely disabled patients may require a spring-lift chair, which must be carefully adjusted according to the user's weight, so that there is no danger of being catapulted out as he rises. Electrically operated chairs of various designs may be appropriate. In some only the seat rises, in others seat and arms rise and in others the whole chair rises. In many the seat tilts forward as well as rising.

The patient should be instructed in rising from a chair correctly, to minimize stress on the joints. He should move forward a little on the seat, place one foot a little in front of the other, grasp the chair arms, keeping the hands pointing forwards, lean slightly forward and rise.

Patients should be discouraged from piling cushions into chairs. They detract from the arm height, making rising more difficult, and soft seats impede rising. If an otherwise suitable chair sags in the seat, a board cut to size may be placed on it, and a slim cushion placed on top. A low chair is better raised from below, so the proportions of the chair are unaffected and it is more stable than cushioning. Standard methods of raising chairs include raising blocks, sleeves and frames. A platform may be constructed as a one-off, but must be designed and constructed by a competent technician in order that the patient is not put at risk. Other accessories include a small bead cushion to support the lumbar or cervical spine. Tripillows or L-shaped cushioning are contra-indicated, as they encourage rounded shoulders and crowded chests. A footstool is unnecessary if the seat height is correct. It is difficult to place and may present a hazard.

Should office seating be required, assessment follows similar lines with easy adjustability being a priority:

- well padded fabric upholstery;
- seat angle adjustable from level to 10° downward, to avoid pressure behind the knees;
- seat height adjustable, to suit task being undertaken;
- backrest adjustable for height and angle;
- armrests optional, about 11 inches (28 cm) long, to get close enough to desk;
- five star base for stability, with glides being safer than castors on uncarpeted floor.

Personal activities of daily living

Toileting may present serious difficulties. Possible solutions include:

- raised toilet seat and/or frame, or combination aid;
- handrails on walls beside toilet cause less strain on arthritic upper limbs;
- spring-lift toilet seat. Precautions as for spring-lift chair;
- ladies may find a loop attached to the inside skirt hem helpful, to be held in the teeth while adjusting the clothing;
- bottom wiper/sponge on an angled handle for hygiene purposes, with built-up handle if necessary;
- ideally, provision of a bidet or clos-o-mat.

Bathing problems are common and solutions include:

- essential provision of non-slip bath or shower mat;
- bath board and seat are standard provision by community agencies. If lowering into the bath, there is stress on the upper limbs when getting up and down;
- mangar type of bath aid avoids stress on upper limbs and enables patient to get right down into water;
- handrails in strategic positions on wall, across bath or outer side of bath;
- special chunky waste plug;
- lever or adapted taps;
- ideally, step-in or walk-in shower, but expensive to install;
- handrail and shower seat also needed;

- long-handled sponge, long flannel with tape loops either end, or a washing mitt with soap pocket;
- bath robe as alternative to towel.

Grooming is important as it detracts from any deformity. Padded, lengthened or angled handles on combs, toothbrushes, make-up equipment, etc., Stirex scissors, toothpaste squeezers and mirrors placed at strategic angles all help in this respect. It may help if the elbows are supported on a table or worktop to perform these tasks.

Dressing is more easily done while seated and resting the elbows on the dressing table may help to get clothes over the head. It is also helpful to choose:

- garments a size larger than needed;
- lightweight clothing in knitted fabrics, in natural fibres for comfort;
- clothes with few fastenings, any fastenings being at the front, using velcro, large buttons and large tabs on zip-pulls;
- elastic waistbands, shoelaces and elasticated or clip-on ties.

Tools likely to help with dressing include:

- dressing stick;
- button hook;
- long reacher, with forearm extension if wrist is unstable;
- long shoehorn;
- sock or tights aid. If the patient is on steroids or has thin shiny skin, the skin on the shins may be damaged by a gutter type aid. The Brevetti type is safer.

Obtaining comfortable footwear is a major problem. Surgical footwear is only prescribed if the patient's needs cannot be met by purchasing standard shoes. 'Off-the-peg' orthopaedic shoes are available from several specialist firms; details are listed in the *Disabled Living Foundation Handbook*, Section 14. These shoes are lightweight, broad, with a deep toe space and available with velcro fastenings. Shoes may be made on the individual's own last, giving a perfect fit until further joint changes occur. There should be no hard toecaps and materials should be suede or very soft leather, with felt for some indoor shoes although this gives little support.

When buying shoes, both feet should be measured while standing and the shoes fitted while wearing any insoles or other appliances normally worn. It is better to buy shoes late in the day, as the feet tend to swell as the day wears on. If the shoe is to be adapted, it is wise to check that they can be changed if the technician finds them unsuitable. Solid heels are needed for fitting calipers. If metatarsalgia or calcaneal spurs are present, plastazote insoles can be fitted by the occupational therapist. Lace up or velcro fastenings give better support.

Buckles are awkward to fasten. If a patient has to wear boots for instability at the ankle joint, a wooden or polypropylene boot remover may be useful.

Because many patients find the weight of the bedclothes over the feet intolerable, a bed cradle may be required.

Eating and drinking tools may be necessary. Patients should try several types of adapted cutlery to find that best suited to their needs. Generally, thick handles are most appropriate, angled towards the mouth. The handles should be shaped to accommodate any deformity, or have the thicker part of the handle on the ulnar side of the hand. Cutlery should be as unobtrusive as possible, especially if the patient eats in company. Cups and mugs must be lightweight, preferably with two handles, or the second hand should be used to support the cup, to prevent the fingers being forced into ulnar deviation. A plate with a deep inward curved rim helps in the control of food and is more acceptable than a plate guard. Dycem matting holds the plate still.

Housing adaptations

For many rheumatoid patients a bungalow or ground floor flat would be ideal, but often an existing house has to be adapted. It is preferable for a patient to remain in his own locality, where he is more likely to have friends and support. If a transfer is essential for the patient's safety, the social worker negotiates for this and the occupational therapist may be asked to write a supporting letter. Warden-controlled accommodation provides security and a suitably appointed home, but there are few younger neighbours to provide stimulation and help and, as the population around is elderly, the frequency of funerals can be depressing. If younger people have to move home, they are likely to miss the support of old friends. They also have to consider proximity to their workplace and possible disruption of their children's education if they have to change school.

If the patient is to remain in his existing home, necessary adaptations may include the following:

- uneven paths relaid and handrails provided, especially if there are steps or slopes;
- grabrails on the door frame, at the optimum height for the patient's use, bearing in mind the limitations imposed by arthritic shoulders;
- draught excluders at the threshold replaced by flexible type attached to base of door;
- a shallow porch with a second front door make access difficult;
- automatically opening garage doors. Up-and-over doors strain the shoulders;
- doors may need adaptation to allow walking frame or wheelchair access. Sliding or folding doors, a door rehung to open outwards or on the opposite

side of the frame may facilitate access;
- lever type door handles;
- furniture arranged to allow plenty of circulation space if walking frame or wheelchair used;
- short-pile carpets make for easier mobility. Avoid loose mats;
- high level controls necessary on gas and electric fires. Central heating on a time-switch is ideal. District Council grants may be available for installation of central heating. Gas and Electricity Boards will adapt controls to enable easier operation. Outside help is needed if solid fuel heating is used;
- stairs may be difficult, especially if steep or winding. A second handrail provides extra security and support, but the patient should not put stress on the arms by hauling himself up;
- a stair or through-floor lift may be necessary. This entails skilled assessment with the lift company concerned. Provision is usually through the Social Services department and may take many weeks due to assessment and committee procedures. Local councils may make a grant towards installation;
- if there is a downstairs toilet and bathroom, bringing the bed downstairs should be a short-term solution only. This situation fosters the invalid role and does not promote quality of life;
- if a new toilet is installed, it should be raised on a plinth;
- a separate shower to replace the bath;
- for a patient living alone, an emergency alarm system may be advisable. To afford legitimate callers access, a two-way communication may be wired up to the door bell.

The grant system for housing adaptations does change from time to time. If a patient is on Income Support, adaptations are carried out free of charge, otherwise assistance is means-related. In some cases an Environmental Health grant is 'topped up' by Social Services. The procedure is slow and ponderous and patients may have to wait many months, sometimes up to two years, for adaptations. The occupational therapist must therefore make satisfactory temporary arrangements.

Household tasks

The occupational therapist should enquire as to what help the patient has at home. The amount the patient undertakes should depend on his physical condition, with adaptation being continuous as the disease progresses and as life tasks alter. The ability to adapt enables the patient to maintain the maximum possible independence. Patient and therapist together should plan the week's activity, spacing out the more arduous tasks and deciding which the patient would be willing to omit altogether and which could be allocated to a helper.

With regard to kitchen activities, the following suggestions put into practice the principles of joint protection and energy conservation:

- use of lightweight saucepans, bowls, etc.;
- filling kettle from a plastic jug and using minimum amount of water necessary;
- jug kettle is lighter than traditional kettle and can be tilted instead of lifted;
- use of kettle and/or teapot tipper when pouring;
- use of wire saucepan basket in pan to make straining of vegetables an automatic process, leaving the water in the pan;
- split level cooker and adapted control knobs;
- electric can openers are indispensable. Different types should be tried before purchase;
- the Rex vegetable peeler with its wide grip is popular;
- serrated or scalloped blade knives are rated more highly by patients with rheumatoid arthritis than the ergonomically shaped knife, with handle at right angles to the blade.
- electric carving knives are heavy, therefore less useful;
- potatoes may be washed and boiled in their skins to save work and preserve nutritional value;
- patients should try a variety of bottle and jar openers to find the one best suited to them;
- use of a stabilizer such as the Belliclamp;
- if an electric mixer is used, it must be on a stand;
- use of electric plugs with handles;
- lever type or adapted water taps;
- keep to simple recipes and procedures.

If no car is available, shopping should be done frequently, so that there is little to carry, and should be carried in a bag across the shoulders, in a trolley or a small bag in each hand.

Heavy cleaning is to be avoided, but dusting and polishing using a sheepskin polishing mitt is beneficial exercise. If stairs are a problem, the patient should ensure that upstairs chores are done before coming down in the morning. An automatic washing machine with a tumble dryer is a boon. When hand washing, the patient must not wring out the clothes. A potato masher will press out a lot of water, ready for the washing to go in the spin dryer. Easy-care fabrics should be chosen as far as possible and only the bare minimum of ironing done, sitting on a perching stool to rest the legs. Bedmaking is much easier if duvets are used, although help will be needed when changing the cover. Moving cleaning materials and other items around on a trolley saves energy.

Holding scissors with the index finger ahead of the loop gives more control

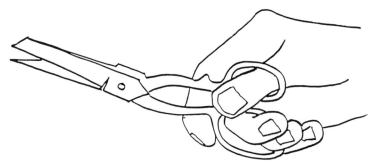

Figure 1.3 Method of manipulating scissors

and less discomfort (Figure 1.3). Stirex type scissors are lightweight and do not aggravate the thumb joints, but are not efficient at cutting through thicker cloth.

Very occasionally, environmental control equipment, such as POSSUM, will be needed and in the event of this, the suppliers of the equipment employ staff to assess and instruct the patient. Intercom systems are frequently used and are easily operated.

Hoists are sometimes required for the handling of severely disabled patients, needing careful assessment and instruction in use. Unless the occupational therapist is assessing for such equipment regularly, it is advisable to turn to an expert for help, with the Disabled Living Centre as the first point of contact.

Communication

If the fingers or thumb of the dominant hand are stiff or painful, a padded pen or one with a moulded holder may be helpful. Finger yokes or pens pushed through a rubber ball may be easier to hold. It is harmful for the patient to write for long because of the static muscle action.

Useful telephone adaptations include large push buttons and a holder, so that the hand is not in a static position while holding the handset.

Sexual problems

Various elements in arthritis (or any other physical disability) contribute to emotional and sexual problems. Such elements include physical appearance, negative body image, pain, loss of or abnormality of function and the effect of drugs. This may lead to the individual feeling unattractive to the opposite sex, where even the development of a friendship is hampered, let alone a flirtation or courtship. Because emotional relationships are so vitally important, this problem must be addressed, and certain staff, including occupational therapists, may develop special counselling skills in this area.

Comparatively few patients of childbearing age will be encountered but their needs will differ from the sexual needs later in life. Contraception is a matter for the general practitioner or family planning clinic to advise on as to the best method for the individual. The couple must consider whether they can cope with the demands of bringing up a family.

The subject of sexual relationships applies to single people as well as to couples and is not an easy one to address. If one looks in the nursing profile under 'expressing sexuality', invariably one finds that the nurse has written 'not discussed'. There has been a tendency to regard people with disabilities as sexless, although their needs are becoming more recognized. If the occupational therapist feels unable to advise on such matters, she must be sure to know to whom to refer the patient who needs advice. The patient must be aware that he can obtain help in this respect, although the decision to seek help should be left to him. Discreet alternatives are to have the address of the Sexual and Personal Relationships of the Disabled (S.P.O.D.) organization on a poster in the department, or to supply an information pack to the patient containing a copy of *Arthritis: Sexual Aspects and Parenthood* published by the Arthritis and Rheumatism Council.

If the arthritis existed pre-maritally, or if both partners are disabled, fewer problems may arise. There are various manifestations of sexual disability for the arthritis sufferer. Deformity makes a person feel less physically attractive and fear of rejection causes anxiety, with the knock-on effect of impotence or frigidity. Depression, fear, pain and medication may suppress the sex drive. Deformed hands may make foreplay difficult. Pain in the woman's hips may make it uncomfortable for her to bear her partner's weight, and pain in the man's arms may make it painful to take weight on them, if the traditional position is adopted. An arthritic husband who has lost his breadwinner role and who has sexual difficulties suffers loss of manhood. Other situations drain energy that might be directed towards sex: due to her husband's arthritis, the wife has to be the breadwinner and housewife: the wife with arthritis struggling to manage home and family: the wife has arthritis and is severely disabled, so the husband has to be breadwinner and do domestic chores, etc.

The couple should be encouraged to discuss their problems together and to find mutually acceptable solutions. An analgesic taken shortly before intercourse, or a change of position, may solve the problem. Depending on which partner has arthritis, and which joints are worst affected, alternative positions may be attempted, such as the woman lying on top of the man, the couple lying on their sides with the man entering from behind, or the man sitting on a chair with the woman sitting astride him. Where it is not possible to achieve intercourse, the couple might indulge in caressing, stroking, kissing, etc., and even lying close together in bed may give them the sense of closeness they need.

Hobbies

While a feature of rheumatoid arthritis is fatigue and sufferers require frequent rest periods, it is important to remember that their minds are still active and they may wish for the company of others with similar interests. Even the person who is content to watch television may need adaptations to the controls. Creative writing or painting are possible hobbies to encourage, with the likelihood of having to modify the pen or brush. Various craft activities are valuable in maintaining function and some local authorities employ craft instructors for people with disabilities. For those who enjoy reading, a book holder is needed so that the hand joints are not stressed.

The person with arthritis should be encouraged in the pursuit of an interest and possibly belong to a club. Some organizations cater specifically for his needs, among them Arthritis Care, who also run several holiday hotels (see also Chapter 12).

Travel

For many patients with arthritis, the car is their link with the outside world. A transfer board may solve any difficulty in getting in and out of the car, or a swivel car seat can be fitted. A two-door car is easier to enter than a four-door, as the doors are wider. There are cars on the market which accommodate a wheelchair-bound driver, but they are expensive. Back supports may be required and should be sampled in the patient's car before purchase. Correctly adjusted head restraints protect against whiplash injury in the event of a bump, and extra mirrors may be needed if the patient's neck is affected. Automatic gears, power-assisted steering and servo-assisted brakes are desirable. Alteration to hand controls, adaptations to the handbrake, steering wheel knobs, etc. are available. Several driving associations (addresses in appendix) give advice on all aspects of driving.

If mobility is appreciably restricted, the patient must be told how to obtain an 'orange badge', entitling him to park in restricted or prohibited places, for ease of access to shops, bank, etc. (see also Chapter 12).

A person whose mobility is severely affected and who is under retirement age should be given a form to apply for Mobility Allowance from the Department of Social Security. He will be assessed by an independent doctor before this is granted. The money may be used to travel by taxi, to maintain his own car, or to acquire a car on the Motability Scheme (see Chapter 12 for details). People with rheumatoid arthritis possessing Department of Social Security vehicles must be medically assessed annually to ensure that they are still fit to drive.

Independent mobility using a car is especially important when we consider public transport. Although most buses designate the front few seats for the use of the elderly or disabled people, a person with rheumatoid disease may find it difficult to grasp the handrail, get up the step or tuck his feet safely away once seated. Travel by underground has other problems: congestion, long distances to walk. Rail travel, unless accompanied, is daunting: narrow difficult steps, formidable gaps between steps and platfrom, unwieldy door handles. If British Rail are notified in advance, staff are helpful in transporting chairbound passengers in good lifts and allowing travel in the guard's van if the traveller cannot get out of the wheelchair. This denies the traveller the dignity he deserves, but this situation is on line for improvement. Airlines, if alerted when the flight is booked, make excellent provision for those with disabilities.

Looking after babies and small children

While pregnant mothers usually have relief from their arthritis symptoms, they may return post-natally. Everything possible should be done by the mother for her child, but if she has to accept help in practical tasks, every effort should be made to ensure that she can cuddle her baby. If there is any danger of the baby being dropped off her knee, he can be fastened into a harness and a walking rein looped over her shoulder to secure him.

Bottlefeeding requires much manual dexterity, so breastfeeding is to be encouraged. The child can then be weaned straight onto baby mugs. Flexible plastic bibs are convenient, as fastening and cleaning them is easy.

Disposable nappies are easier to handle than towelling squares and eliminate the laundry problem. Two major distributors of nappies provide free home delivery. It is important to choose the right sized nappy and those with a long strip allowing adjustment when fastening the self-adhesive tabs are preferable. The baby should be changed on a high surface suited to the mother's height. Once baby grows and becomes stronger, he needs a toy to distract him while being changed. Baby wipes make cleaning easier.

Small babies are easily bathed in the kitchen sink. A baby bath which fits across the normal bath is available and can be filled from a shower head or hose. It has its own waste plug. Otherwise, the mother needs the full bath carrying for her. A baby bath wrap makes for easier drying.

A child born to a parent with arthritis tends to adapt quickly and learns to co-operate. He can be taught to dress himself at an earlier age and to climb up to his parent's level for help. It is important that he recognizes that this is the only time he may climb onto furniture. The type of clothing chosen should be similar to that chosen for the parent.

When the time comes for toilet training, it is easier to use the adaptor seats for normal toilets, with a sturdy box for the child to climb onto the seat.

Baby furniture such as cots, high chairs, prams and pushchairs can present problems in lifting the child in and out, and in operating movable parts. Selection of such items should be done on an individual basis, with regard to the particular difficulties of the parent.

Safety gates are needed to protect the child from the danger of stairs. To enable the baby to be carried more safely on the stairs, there should be a handrail each side and the baby should be held facing forwards with the parent's arm around his body under his arms.

Once the child is toddling, he should be held by reins when on the road. When in parks and playgrounds, he must learn not to run off out of sight and sound of his parent.

Because the parent may be on drugs to control the arthritis, special care must be taken to ensure the child cannot get at them. This is particularly important as the child-proof containers may have been changed to a type more easily opened by the parent.

SUPPORT GROUPS

These may be set up for the mutual support of patients but it may be appropriate to have occasional multidisciplinary professional input. Patients are able to air their frustrations concerning the effects of their illness and their fears of future incapacitation. They can discuss their practical problems and learn how others solve theirs. They can also exchange experiences about community resources, local facilities and leisure interests. If a professional is present, her role is to listen, then perhaps suggest solutions to problems and correct any misapprehensions which have become evident. These groups may also be involved in campaigning in such matters as local access, benefits, etc.

ANKYLOSING SPONDYLITIS

Ankylosing spondylitis is the chief of the seronegative arthroses. It differs from rheumatoid arthritis in that the rheumatoid factor is absent, the sacro-iliac joints and spine are involved, joint inflammation is asymmetrical, more than five times as many men as women are affected, and iritis occurs and may lead to visual impairment.

The onset tends to occur in the early twenties and starts in the sacro-iliac joints then progresses up the lumbar spine into the thoracic and cervical spine. The attachments of the ligaments to the bones become inflamed, then heal by forming small knobs of new bone. Eventually the whole ligament becomes bone and results in the development of the 'bamboo spine'. The typical deformity is of a round-shouldered man, sometimes bowed almost at right angles to the legs, while the cervical spine may be extended so that he can look ahead.

The pain and stiffness are relieved by exercise but aggravated by rest, especially when in bed. Bending and twisting become increasingly difficult, as does turning the head. The pain ceases once rigidity has occurred. If both spine and hips stiffen, walking and sitting become very difficult.

Treatment concentrates on correcting the posture, with physiotherapy to maintain mobility of all spinal joints plus breathing exercises, with exercise periods twice daily. Swimming is encouraged, as back stroke is excellent therapy, with breast stroke providing specific exercise for shoulder and hip joints, and front crawl to exercise the spine. Diving and contact sports are contra-indicated. Analgesia and anti-inflammatory drugs are prescribed.

If the spine has not already fused, the maintenance of good posture ensures that, when fusion does occur, it will be in a good functional position. To this end a firm mattress should be used, without a pillow. If this last is intolerable, one slim pillow is permitted. The armchair should have a high, firm backrest, supporting the whole spine including the cervical spine. Sitting for any length of time is not tolerated. If the hips have ankylosed, a saddle type seat may be required for a working chair and a recliner for an armchair. Office seating is needed as for rheumatoid arthritis, plus padded armrests as these patients tend to use their forearms when changing position.

The most likely surgery for these patients is hip replacement. Occasionally corrective spinal osteotomy is performed, aimed at straightening the spine.

The National Ankylosing Spondylitis Society funds research into the disease and provides education and information for the patient on a wide range of topics (address in appendix).

REFERENCES

Disabled Living Foundation (1988) *Information Service Handbook* (Section 14: Footwear), Disabled Living Foundation, London.

Furst, G.P., Gerber, L.H. and Smith, C.B. (1985) *Rehabilitation Through Learning: Energy conservation and joint protection – a workbook for persons with rheumatoid arthritis*, US Govt Printing Office, Washington DC

Greengross, W. *Arthritis: Sexual aspects and parenthood*, Arthritis and Rheumatism Council, Chesterfield.

Souter, W.A. (1987) Surgical management of rheumatoid arthritis, in S.P.F. Hughes, M.K Benson and C. Colton (eds.) *Orthopaedics: The principles and practice of musculoskeletal surgery*, Churchill Livingstone, Edinburgh.

Spiegel, J.S., Hirshfield, M.S. and Spiegel, T.S. (1985) Evaluating self-care activities; comparison of a self-reported questionnaire with an occupational therapist interview, *British Journal of Rheumatology*, **24**, 357–61.

FURTHER READING

Atherton, J., Chatfield, J., Clarke, A.K. and Harrison, R.A. (1979) *Easy Chairs for the Arthritic*, DHSS Aids Assessment Programme, DHSS.

Atherton, J., Clarke, A.K. and Harrison, R.A. (1981) *Office Seating for the Arthritic and Low Back Pain Patients*, DHSS Aids Assessment Programme, DHSS.

Baker, G.H.B. (1981) Psychological management of the patient with rheumatoid arthritis, *Clinics in Rheumatic Diseases*, 7, no. 2, 455–67.

Bradshaw, E.S.R. (1985) *Food Preparation Aids for Rheumatoid Arthritis Patients, Part 2A*, DHSS Aids Assessment Programme, DHSS.

Brattstrom, M. (1973) *Principles of Joint Protection in Chronic Rheumatic Disease*, Wolfe Medical Books, London.

Caruso, L.A. *et al.* A.H.P.A. Task Force (1986) Roles and functions of occupational therapy in the management of patients with rheumatic diseases, *American Journal of Occupational Therapy*, 40, no. 12, 825–9.

Clarke, A., Allard, L. and Braybrooks, B. (1987) *Rehabilitation in Rheumatology: The team approach*, Martin Dunitz, London.

Furst, G.P., Gerber, L.H., Smith, C.C., Fisher, S. and Shulman, B. (1987) A programme for improving energy conservation behaviours in adults with rheumatoid arthritis, *American Journal of Occupational Therapy*, 41, no. 2, 102–11.

Melvin, J.L. (1980) *Rheumatic Disease: Occupational therapy and rehabilitation*, F.A. Davis, Philadelphia.

Nichols, P.J.R. *et al.* (1980) *Rehabilitation Medicine: The management of physical disabilities*, 2nd Edn, Butterworths, London.

Orford, J. (1987) *Coping with Disorder in the Family*, Croom Helm, London.

Panayi, G.S. (1980) *Essential Rheumatology for Nurses and Therapists*, Baillière Tindall, London.

Pedretti, L.W. (1980) *Occupational Therapy Practice Skills for Physical Dysfunction*, Mosby, St Louis.

Salter, M. (1988) *Altered Body Image*, Wiley, Chichester.

Trombly, C. (1983) *Occupational Therapy for Physical Dysfunction*, 2nd edn, Williams and Wilkins, Baltimore.

Wilshere, E.R., Cochrane, G.M. and O'Brien, P.M. (1989) *Parents with Disabilities*. Equipment for Disabled People Series, Oxfordshire Health Authority, Oxford.

2

Total hip replacement

This is probably the operation most associated with orthopaedic wards. It is also one of the most quoted when hospital waiting lists are under discussion. It is mainly the elderly who need hip replacement and, with increased longevity and the expectation of better quality of life, this surgery is in ever-increasing demand. Improving techniques and prostheses allow younger people to have hip replacements, adding to the demand.

REASONS FOR TOTAL HIP REPLACEMENT

Hip replacement is most often prescribed for primary osteo-arthritis, which is the process of joint degeneration in the elderly. It is colloquially referred to as 'wear and tear', but there is no obvious cause of this. The process starts with weakening and destruction of the cartilage. The underlying bone becomes hard and sometimes cystic. In the advanced stages there is complete loss of cartilage from large areas of the joint surface (**eburnation**). New bone forms at the joint margins (**osteophytes**) and the joint becomes fibrosed.

Secondary osteo-arthritis follows some obvious predisposing cause, e.g. congenital dislocation of the hip, acetabular dysplasia, Perthes' disease, rheumatoid arthritis, trauma or infection of the joint.

Pain and stiffness are first felt when rising after a period of rest. This becomes progressively worse until the patient finds it hard to bend down to put on his socks or cut his toenails. Limping may be noticed early. Internal rotation, abduction and extension are the first movements to be lost. If a fixed deformity develops the leg lies in external rotation and adduction and therefore appears short. This also causes a limp. Patients present with pain in the groin. Pain may also be felt in the buttock, over the greater trochanter and down the leg to just above the knee. This is because the hip and knee are supplied by the same nerves.

OUTLINE OF SURGERY

The Charnley low-friction arthroplasty has stood the test of time. It consists of a stainless steel femoral component and a high density polyethylene acetabular cup,

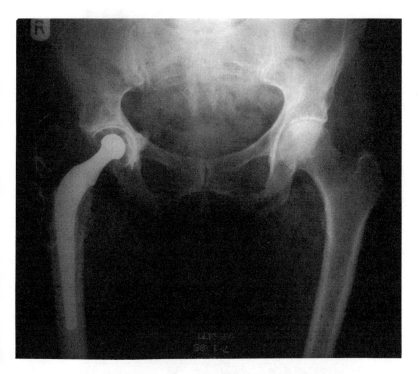

Figure 2.1 Charnley total hip replacement, showing broken wires with displacement of greater trochanter

each fixed with methylmethacrylate bone cement to give greater bonding power. The cement hardens within a few minutes, so fixation is secure very quickly.

During the operation the head and part of the neck of the femur are removed. The greater trochanter used to be removed and replaced after the prosthesis was in place (Figure 2.1), but this has been largely discontinued and the greater trochanter may be left in situ throughout. The greatest threat to the operation is infection and in order to guard against this, the operation is performed within a 'Charnley tent' or other ultra-clean-air system. Antibiotics are usually employed as an additional precaution.

Complications following hip replacement include deep vein thrombosis and the warning sign of this may be pain in the calf. This may lead to pulmonary embolism. Very occasionally the femoral shaft fractures during surgery and, even more rarely, the acetabulum fractures.

Continuing developments include the use of components with perforations or porous coatings into which the bone grows, eliminating the need for cement (Figure 2.2). The thinking behind this is that there is less chance of the prosthesis

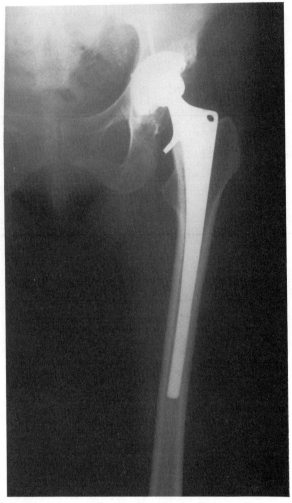

Figure 2.2 Total hip replacement; Harris Galante cup with bias stem, uncemented

loosening, but this is debatable. This technique can be useful for younger patients but the patient must be non-weightbearing for a period post-operatively. If the prosthesis does not become secure over its total surface, or becomes infected, the revision surgery can be more difficult.

The Exeter system consists of a collarless, double-tapered, wedge design of femoral stem, with a choice of femoral head and acetabular cup. An intramedullary plug at the distal end of the femoral component prevents bone cement migrating into the intramedullary canal. As it engages, the tapered design transmits load through the cement to the bone, ensuring a tight fit and a reduction in shear stress, aimed at reducing the incidence of loosening.

PRE-OPERATIVE OCCUPATIONAL THERAPY

Because of the possibility of having to revise the surgery later, the joint is allowed to degenerate considerably prior to surgery. Meanwhile analgesics, anti-inflammatory drugs and physiotherapy are used. The patient is provided with a stick to relieve weightbearing and is asked to limit his weightbearing activity. Because patients with arthritic hips have problems with activities of daily living (ADL), occupational therapy intervention is indicated whether or not the patient is to undergo surgery.

Increasingly, hospitals are undertaking pre-operative assessment of patients on a day-patient basis to ensure that the patient is fit for surgery on admission. The patient is X-rayed, has blood tests, blood pressure check, electrocardiogram, urine test and is checked to exclude dental decay, ulcers or other potential sources of infection. The surgery is explained and admission normally follows within two to three weeks. The patient meets the physiotherapist and the occupational therapist who explain their respective roles so that the patient understands and accepts the reason for all the questions asked of him. These questions include the following:

1. Does the patient live alone? If with a carer, is the carer fit?
2. Does he live in a house, bungalow or flat?
3. If in a flat, is there a lift?
4. Is the accommodation owner-occupied, council or privately rented property? This is relevant when requesting adaptations to property.
5. Where is the toilet? If downstairs, is it indoors? If outside, is there a covered way to reach it; are there steps to negotiate?
6. Where is the bathroom? Is there a separate shower? Are any bathing aids in situ?
7. Is there at least one sturdy stair-rail?
8. Does the patient sleep upstairs?
9. Is the bed firm and high enough to rise from, i.e. 20–24 inches from floor to top of mattress, depending on patient's height?
10. Has he an armchair from which he can rise easily?
11. Has he any aids to enable easy rising from the toilet?
12. Does he wear slip-on or lace-up shoes?
13. Question for ladies: are tights or stockings worn?
14. Does he normally have help with cooking or housework?
15. Can meals be taken in the kitchen? If not, is there level access from kitchen to living room?
16. What commitments does he have to family, work, other?

Armed with the above information, the occupational therapist gets a picture of the patient in his home setting and can requisition necessary equipment from community agencies. The patient must be instructed in the safe and correct use of any tools supplied and all equipment must be fitted by a competent person. Equipment which may be required includes:

- raised toilet seat, suited to the patient's height;
- toilet frame or handrails on wall;
- high seat chair or raising devices;
- bed raising devices;
- long reaching tool;
- long shoehorn;
- stocking or tights gutter;
- elastic shoelaces;
- trolley to transport meals from kitchen to living room;
- bath board and seat (these are usually regarded as low priority by community agencies).

It is useful to give the patient a handout summarizing what has transpired as a reminder, as he will be bombarded with information at this pre-operative assessment.

Alternatively, the patient may be referred to the occupational therapy department as soon as he goes onto the waiting list. He then attends for assessment as above, or if staffing levels permit, a home assessment is carried out. If the latter, the therapist can assess suitability of chairs, etc. at first hand without having to depend on the patient's sometimes doubtful descriptions. Patients are thus enabled to cope more comfortably in the time running up to their surgery. Generally the onus should be on the patient to obtain a suitable chair and bed and advice concerning these items should be given. In cases of real need, referral may be made to community agencies and a social worker, and information given concerning benefits available.

POST-OPERATIVE MANAGEMENT

Prior to surgery the patient is allowed to perform any movement of which he is capable. Following surgery, healing must take place in the soft tissues to provide stability. It is possible to dislocate the new hip while the soft tissues are still weak. Opinions differ depending on the individual surgeon and the surgical approach, but a general rule is to take precautions for three months post-operatively.

In order to prevent dislocation, the hip movements which the patient must avoid are adduction, flexion beyond 90° and rotation. Usually a 'Charnley wedge' or a fat pillow is placed between the legs while lying in bed, to prevent these movements. Patients are normally up on the second post-operative day. The physiotherapist oversees the walking and general mobility. She teaches the patient to rise from bed, chair and toilet by sliding the operated leg forward, then taking the weight on the arms, sliding forward in the chair (avoiding wriggling forward) and rising without flexing the trunk onto the thighs, taking the strain on the unoperated leg. To sit down this procedure is reversed.

Authorities disagree about which side of the bed the patient should get in and out. Generally the patient is taught to get in and out on the operated side as there is a reduced chance of adduction of the operated leg. What is more important is to ensure that there is no adduction across the midline of the body, no rotation and no flexion beyond 90°.

Weightbearing on the new hip is commenced at once, using a walking frame and progressing to two sticks within a few days as the patient gains stability and confidence. Just before discharge the physiotherapist teaches the technique of stair management. The rule for this is easily remembered: 'Good up to heaven, bad down to hell', i.e. the good (unoperated) leg leads going upstairs and the bad (operated) leg leads going downstairs. The following leg is brought up to the first but not past it, in the manner of a young child negotiating stairs.

OCCUPATIONAL THERAPY

Aims:

- to enable the patient to be independent in ADL;
- to promote healing and restore muscle power;
- to encourage a positive attitude and gradual return to a normal lifestyle.

Objectives: following instruction by the occupational therapist and practice in a safe environment, the patient will be able to:

- perform all necessary activities of daily living with use of appropriate tools;
- understand how to protect his prosthesis, supported by a written list of 'do's and don'ts';
- perform gentle activity within the prescribed limits.

The flow chart (Figure 2.3) is a convenient method for monitoring the achievement of objectives, particularly useful if a collaborative care planning system is in operation. Collaborative care planning is a multidisciplinary approach to the assessment and management of an episode of care, in collaboration with the patient. Its purpose is effective use of resources by the clear planning, implementation and monitoring of the total treatment package. Pre-admission screening, objectives, daily care plans, post-discharge follow-up and clinical audit are included in the plan, and the paperwork for each discipline is open-plan on the clipboard at the foot of the patient's bed. If the patient has already been

OCCUPATIONAL THERAPY DEPARTMENT T.H.R.

NAME:

NUMBER:

DATE:

Pre-Op	Op.	Day 1	Day 2	Day 3	Day 4	Day 5	Day 6	Day 7	Day 8	Day 9	Day 10	Day 11	Day 12	Day 13 etc
Assess home situation accom., help,aids already supplied		loan h/hand	As Pre-Op (if not already done)	→	↗									
						Access for toilet aids	→	↗						
								Teach use of dressing aids	Monitor	→	↗			
								Order necessary equipment	→	↗				
									Kitchen practice if appropriate	→	↗			
											Confirm Discharge date to supplying agency when known	Check equipment delivered and fitted		
					Observe correct movement patterns	→	↗							Home visit for high risk patients
														→

Figure 2.3 Flow chart for monitoring achievement of objectives following T.H.R.

assessed and instructed during the pre-admission screening, the objectives on the chart will be modified accordingly.

It is important that the patient does not sit in a deep, low chair. If a high chair is not available, an existing chair should be adapted by raising from beneath so as not to alter the balance of the chair, using Langham raisers, sleeves or blocks. With these last, it is necessary to place the chair against a wall for stability, in case the chair moves back as the patient sits down. Piles of cushions make the seat too soft to rise from and may cause the hips to rotate, thus risking dislocation. They also take up space so that the full benefit of the arms of the chair are not felt when rising. Only one extra cushion should be placed on the seat, and that a slim one, with a board beneath it to provide a firmer base. A Putnam wedge will comfortably adapt a carver chair. A pillow may be placed at the back of a deep chair to hold the patient forward.

Some swelling of the foot and lower leg is usual for a few weeks after surgery due to congestion of the veins in the leg. The leg must be kept up when at rest, the foot level with the hip, and the ankle regularly rotated 20 times in each direction to encourage contraction of gastrocnemius and soleus, assisting venous return by the pumping action of the muscles. To avoid overflexion at the hip, the patient should lean back a little in the seat. Later, when the swelling has subsided, he should sit with the knees slightly lower than the hips.

The patient's bed at home may need raising with Langham or St Helier raisers or similar. The height of the top of the mattress from the floor should be higher than the armchair seat, as he has to rise without the assistance of armrests. Depending on the patient's height, 20–24 inches (51–61 cm) is a good height for the bed. If the mattress is soft, a board should be placed under at least the middle of it and preferably under its whole length. Rarely does a patient alter his bedroom layout after surgery, so he may get in and out of bed on the opposite side from when he was in hospital, but he must follow the same basic method. Only very occasionally it is necessary to turn the bed round. The patient should sleep on his back with a pillow between his legs to prevent turning over in his sleep. Later, after discussion with his surgeon, he may lie on his side, again with a pillow between the legs to prevent the uppermost leg crossing the midline.

Most patients require only a raised toilet seat to make them independent in the toilet, the height of the seat depending on the patient's height. Occasionally a toilet frame is also needed, or a combined frame and raised seat. The method of getting up and down as taught in hospital is followed. To flush the toilet, the patient should either turn towards the unoperated side to do so, or he must avoid spinning round on the operated leg, instead taking small steps to turn round to face the flush handle.

Bathing is risky and unless the patient already has suitable bathing equipment, it is wiser to refrain from bathing until three months post-operatively. Pedretti (1981) and Trombly (1983) advocate getting into the bath side-on, lifting the leg over the side by bending the knee. This depends on the height of the bath or the length of leg of the patient in question. The favoured method in Britain is to use a bath board, sitting on it and leaning back slightly to avoid overflexion of the hip, then lifting the leg carefully over the side of the bath. Showering is then possible while sitting on the board, or the patient may move down onto a bath seat. It is inadvisable to sit on the floor of the bath, as the hip is already flexed to 90°. Any reaching to manipulate taps or plug, or washing the feet, overflexes the hip. The feet may be washed using a long-handled sponge or a sponge held in a reaching tool. Use of a separate shower is safer, using a non-slip mat. The patient must not bend to wash the feet.

Dressing should be performed sitting down. To avoid overflexion of the hip, a reacher should be used, putting the operated leg into pants first. Hosiery must be put on with a tool for the purpose. This requires careful instruction, as many patients find it difficult to master. A helper is needed if anti-embolism stockings are worn. If elastic shoe laces are used, they must not be stretched before tying, and a long shoehorn is essential. The shoe tongue may either be held in place by threading the laces through a small hole punched in it, or by pulling the tongue through to the outside, below the laces.

A dropped object can be picked up with a long reacher or the patient can be taught a safe way of picking items up, provided the other hip is sound. He can steady himself on a sturdy piece of furniture, put his operated leg out behind him, then bend down, taking the strain on the unoperated leg.

A patient living alone, or who looks after another person, needs kitchen practice pre-discharge. Usually making a hot drink and perhaps a piece of toast is sufficient to assess competence in the kitchen, observing the patient's mobility and use of his sticks, including any tendency to leave them behind! The patient can be reminded if he does anything which could cause dislocation, and safety in handling gas or electricity and boiling liquid is checked. Moving a kettle or pan of water is difficult when using two sticks, so the patient must be taught to handle a kettle while holding the stick in the other hand, and to avoid carrying these utensils if possible. He should be instructed to slide pans along work surfaces, but if these are not continuous he must put the pan down on a surface a little ahead of him, take a few steps using his sticks, pick up the pan and move it another stage, etc. Any necessary tools for living should be supplied and, if the therapist is not satisfied that the patient is safe, the assessment should be repeated, perhaps cooking a full meal so that vegetable preparation and tin opening may also be assessed.

Vacuuming and heavy housework should be avoided for the first three months after surgery, but simple cooking, washing up, dusting and polishing while standing and walking around gently are excellent exercise for the hip. Frequently used items should be conveniently sited, as climbing and bending are forbidden. Use of the oven should be confined to times when a helper is at hand, and fires with low controls must be left to a helper. Patients should be advised to sit down for 20 to 30 minutes, then get up and move around for a while, before sitting down again, gradually extending the active period.

To get in and out of a car, the car must be parked away from the kerb to gain the maximum height from ground to seat top. The seat back should recline slightly and a firm cushion or Putnam wedge be placed on the seat if it is low. The seat should be pushed as far back as possible and the window wound right down. The patient should turn his back on the car, hold the door on one side and the door frame on the other, and sit down. He should then pull himself back as far as necessary in order to swing his legs round together to bring them into the car. The procedure should be reversed for getting out. The patient should not drive until the surgeon has approved it at the follow-up clinic.

Sexual activity may be resumed after three months, if lying on the unoperated side with the operated leg resting on a pillow, for either sex. A man may lie on his back with the woman astride him. It is advisable for a woman to wait three to four months before lying on her back for intercourse; then a pillow should be placed to prevent the operated hip being pressed out too far.

THE OUTLOOK FOLLOWING HIP REPLACEMENT

Total hip replacement is a routine operation, but is nevertheless major surgery. Elderly patients take longer to recover, partly because of the length of time it takes to excrete the anaesthetic residue. The period of hospitalization gets ever shorter, but every patient is safely mobile and capable of managing stairs on discharge. Three months later he can expect to bend down more freely. By the time six months have elapsed, he really feels the benefit of surgery and the successful operation achieves 90–95% restoration of function.

RESURFACING TOTAL HIP REPLACEMENT

The acetabulum and articulating surface only of the femoral head are replaced (Figure 2.4). The first attempts at this procedure have been largely abandoned because of early failure. Work is proceeding on a modified form with metal on metal articulation. The thinking behind the technique is that there is no femoral stem to loosen and, if the surgery should fail, revision or conversion to a formal hip replacement can more easily be effected. It is too early for results to be evaluated.

Occupational therapy involvement is similar to that for total hip replacement. It is particularly important to protect the joint in the early post-operative weeks and the patient may not bear weight fully for six weeks or more, and then uses two sticks for a further six weeks.

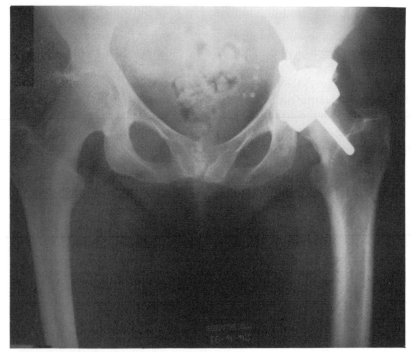

Figure 2.4 Resurfacing total hip replacement, metal on metal components

REVISION OF TOTAL HIP REPLACEMENT

Because of the increasing demand for hip replacement, especially in younger people, there is a corresponding rise in the need for revision surgery. The main reason for revision is loosening of either component. The other reasons for revision are deep infection, recurrent dislocation and fractures. As with primary arthroplasty, pain and loss of function are the criteria for surgery.

When revision is performed, the old prosthesis is removed, the area thoroughly cleaned and every trace of bone cement removed, especially in the case of infection. The operation is considerably more difficult than for primary surgery and the cost very much greater. When the prosthesis is removed, the bone surface is usually smooth and sclerotic, so the bone-cement interface is much less strong in a revision and is reduced still further in any subsequent revision. Bone grafting may be performed if there is loss of bone stock and this entails a much longer period of either bedrest or non-weightbearing postoperatively.

Deep infection is treated with antibiotics, with debridement of the joint and short-term closed suction drainage. If this fails, the implant may be removed and a revision performed using antibiotic-loaded acrylic cement. This is done in one stage if the offending organism is a 'friendly' bug, i.e. one which responds readily to antibiotics. If an 'unfriendly' bug, i.e. one which is more resistant to antibiotics, is the cause of infection, the implant may be removed, then some weeks or months later when it is believed the infection has cleared, the revision is performed. The disadvantages of this latter regime are the cost to the patient, his family and the hospital, risks involved in further surgery and the patient's frustration and incapacitation between the two stages.

Occupational therapy intervention is similar to that for primary surgery, but it is even more important to observe the precautions against dislocation and ensure the patient has all the equipment available to enable him to protect the arthroplasty to get the longest possible life out of it. Because this surgery is tailored to the individual patient, the timescale varies considerably from one to another and the patient's goals are modified accordingly.

REFERENCES

Pedretti, L.W. (1981) *Occupational Therapy Practice Skills for Physical Dysfunction*, Mosby, St Louis.

Trombly, C. (1983) *Occupational Therapy for Physical Dysfunction*, 2nd edn, Williams and Wilkins, Baltimore.

FURTHER READING

Ahnfelt, L., Herberts, P., Malchau, H. and Andersson, G.B.J. (1990) Prognosis of total hip replacement, *Acta Orthop Scand*, **61**, no.238, 9–12.

Browne, P.S.H. (1985) *Basic Facts in Orthopaedics*, 2nd edn, Blackwell Scientific Publications, Oxford.

Fairburn, S.M (1985) Daily activities following hip replacement: a handout, *British Journal of Occupational Therapy*, 48, no.6, 167–8.

Hardinge, K. (1983) *Hip Replacement: The facts*, Oxford University Press, Oxford.

Hughes, S. (1989) *A New Short Textbook of Orthopaedics and Traumatology*, Edward Arnold, London.

Johnson, R., Thorngren, K.G. and Persson, B.M. (1988) Revision of total hip replacement for primary osteoarthritis, *Journal of Bone and Joint Surgery*, **70–B**, no.1, 56–61.

Snorrason, F. and Karrholm, J. (1990) Early loosening of revision hip arthroplasty, *Journal of Arthroplasty*, **5**, no. 3, 217–27.

Steinbrink, K. (1990) The case for revision arthroplasty using antibiotic- loaded acrylic cement, *Clinical Orthopaedics and Related Research*, **261**, 19–22.

3

Other hip surgery

OSTEOTOMY

This is sometimes performed to provide pain relief in the younger patient. One type is the McMurray osteotomy, in which the femur is surgically divided between the greater and lesser trochanters and the shaft of the femur displaced medially, followed by internal fixation with a nail and plate. This redistributes the weightbearing stresses on the joint. Healing takes up to three months. It is frequently a holding operation until joint replacement is carried out later.

Because the hip joint is left intact, the precautions needed following hip replacement are unnecessary. However, depending on the height, build and general fitness of the patient, he may need provision of a raised toilet seat or frame and the occupational therapist should ensure that he can dress his lower half. If the patient's seating at home is low, this should be rectified.

ARTHRODESIS

This operation is less common than it used to be but may be the procedure of choice in younger patients following trauma or septic arthritis. It relieves the hip pain and stabilizes the joint, but a considerable proportion of patients complain of back and knee pain afterwards. The operation involves removal of the remaining cartilage and reshaping the femoral head to fit the acetabulum. A bone graft may be inserted and the whole is internally fixed. A common complication of this procedure is non-union. Patients may be immobilized in a hip spica for three months or longer while healing takes place. The operation causes shortening on the affected side and the patient has then to wear a shoe raise.

Occupational therapy for this patient is essential. At this stage the aims are:

- to enable the patient to be independent in ADL;
- to encourage a positive and adaptive outlook;
- to maintain the maximum activity level possible under the imposed restrictions.

The therapist's assessment should include the same details as for total hip replacement. It is necessary to make both short-term and long-term arrangements for his independence. To enable him to cope at home while wearing the hip spica, the following tools for living may be required:

- raised toilet seat with a dip side to accommodate the hip spica/stiff hip;
- handrail on wall or toilet frame, the latter floor-fixed for stability;

- high commode, with oval-to-round adaptor to accommodate dip side toilet seat raise;
- bedpan and urinal, if above toilet aids not available;
- Femicep toilet aid for female patients;
- bedraising device;
- high seat chair with sloping backrest;
- long reacher;
- long shoehorn.

It is easier for the patient to have his bed downstairs at first, with a commode provided if there is no downstairs toilet. In some households this is a problem, owing to lack of space and privacy. If the patient remains upstairs, he is isolated from family and social contact.

More permanent arrangements are necessary later and, if home conditions warrant it, rehousing may be considered. Once the joint has arthrodesed, the patient can manage stairs by the child's technique already described. Permanent equipment will include:

- a second handrail alongside the stairs;
- provision of a chair with a divided seat, so that the stiff hip is comfortably accommodated and the spine is supported in the optimum position;
- permanent handrails by the toilet;
- long-handled sponge;
- referral to Social Services department for provision of a separate shower.

Car adaptations may be required, e.g. entering the driving seat of a British car will be all right if the left hip is affected, but difficult if the right hip is arthrodesed. The patient should be furnished with all the information he needs to resolve any driving problem.

Sexual activity

The woman with an arthrodesed hip has a problem regarding positioning. She should be given the opportunity to discuss this with an understanding member of staff, or given details of SPOD. Alternative methods of achieving sexual pleasure, such as caressing or sex aids, may be suggested. Some patients may be encouraged and reassured that a professional person has recommended this, since it demonstrates that such methods are acceptable and medically approved.

PELVIC OSTEOTOMY

One technique for osteotomy of the innominate bone is the Chiari osteotomy (Figure 3.1).

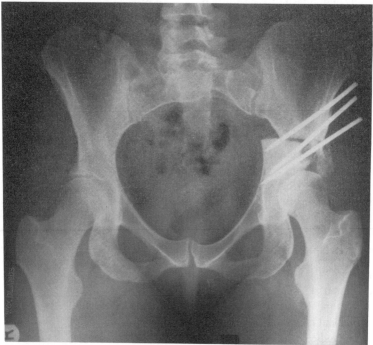

Figure 3.1 Chiari pelvic osteotomy

The procedure is used for younger patients presenting with subluxation or recurrent dislocation of the hip. The operation involves the medial displacement of the distal part of the pelvis, thus deepening the roof of the acetabulum and distributing pressure over a greater area of the head of the femur. Post-operatively, the hip is immobilized in a hip spica, with the hip in 20 – 30° of abduction, for three weeks or more. After removal of plaster, passive and active exercises are commenced and after one more week, partial weightbearing is allowed. The patient may be discharged while wearing the hip spica, and if so the occupational therapist will arrange for equipment to be provided as for short-term provision for the patient with an arthrodesed hip.

This surgery gives better results when performed as primary surgery and on patients where there is little arthritis. A prerequisite is a good range of hip movement. Following surgery there is good correlation between pain relief and function. There may be some shortening, producing a slight limp. If the operation should fail, the improved acetabular bone stock makes total hip replacement easier.

Alternative pelvic osteotomies include the Salter's and shelf operations (Figure 3.2).

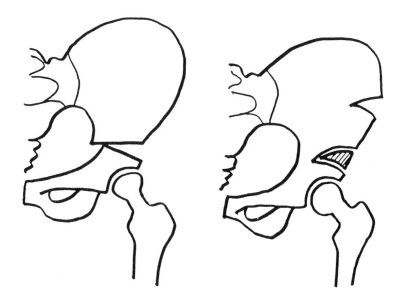

Figure 3.2 Salter's and 'shelf' pelvic osteotomies

GIRDLESTONES EXCISION ARTHROPLASTY

This may be a salvage operation following a failed joint replacement, or a holding operation while awaiting clearance of infection in two stage revision surgery (see p.39) The head and neck of the femur are excised and soft tissue, usually gluteal muscle fibres, is interposed between the acetabulum and femur. This forms a false joint which is painfree and mobile, but unstable (Figure 3.3). The patient requires a walking frame or crutches to mobilize. Some older patients experience difficulty in managing the Girdlestones hip.

Occupational therapy assessment includes the same details as for total hip replacement, but there is no need for precautions against dislocation. Adaptations and tools for living will be needed permanently if the operation is a salvage procedure, and the patient needs items similar to those required following hip replacement. The aims of occupational therapy are as for hip arthrodesis. The objectives are for the patient to:

- perform all necessary ADL tasks safely, using appropriate tools;
- understand and adapt to the imposed physical limitations;
- be safely mobile within these imposed limits.

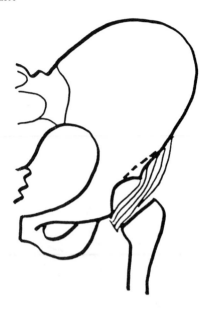

Figure 3.3 Girdlestones excision arthroplasty

CONGENITAL DISLOCATION OF THE HIP

There are a number of procedures for correction of this condition. Early splintage is usual, with the hips held in abduction in a frog plaster for three to six months. The principle behind this treatment is that the maintenance of constant pressure on the femoral head deepens the acetabulum. The child under a year old may have an adductor tenotomy, or a toddler may have a pelvic osteotomy to correct the defective acetabulum. After these operations, immobilization in hip abduction plasters is standard for variable periods of time.

Occupational therapy input is normally only for assessment and requisition of a suitable buggy or wheelchair to accommodate the cumbersome plaster. A suitable car seat may also be required. Because the child is very young, his parents will be attending to his personal needs, but they should be consulted as to any specific difficulties which the occupational therapist can deal with on an ad hoc basis.

A significant proportion of these patients develop secondary arthritis and present later in life for further surgery.

PERTHES' DISEASE

This condition affects children between the ages of three and ten years. Over a period of two to three years, the femoral head becomes denser, after which it appears to fragment, then eventually the bone texture returns to normal. During these changes, deformity of the femoral head and thickening of the neck of femur commonly occur. Subluxation of the hip and secondary arthritis may follow.

The hip is rested with skin traction applied, until the pain and muscle spasm have resolved. A 'broomstick' plaster may then be applied with the hips abducted and internally rotated; this is retained for nine months after which the child is non-weightbearing for approximately 15 months. Alternatively, an innominate (pelvic) osteotomy is performed, when immobilization is for two to three months only.

With regard to occupational therapy, the same applies as for congenital hip dislocation, but as the child is older he needs individual assessment for a wheelchair and for toilet aids. Pants or trousers will need adaptation to fasten along the insides of the legs and crotch.

SLIPPED FEMORAL EPIPHYSIS

This condition is occasionally encountered on the orthopaedic ward. Internal fixation by threaded pins prevents further displacement and stimulates epiphyseal fusion if the condition is treated early (Hughes, 1989). If displacement is considerable, a wedge may be removed from the femoral neck to prevent stretching soft tissue attachments of the displaced epiphysis, or a subtrochanteric osteotomy may be performed. Occupational therapy intervention is unlikely to be necessary.

While the juvenile conditions mentioned are not exhaustive, they do represent the most usual methods of treatment of hip disorders in the very young, which will require occupational therapy intervention.

FEMORAL FRACTURES

Fractures of the femur belong in the field of trauma but may be encountered on the orthopaedic ward. These fractures may be caused by direct or twisting force, osteoporosis or bone tumour.

Osteoporosis is a decrease in bone density, the bone becoming porous and rarified with an increased risk of fractures. The causes are mainly:

- post-menopausal hormone changes;
- old age, i.e. over 65 years;
- immobility;
- prolonged use of corticosteroids.

Less common causes include nutritional deficiency, osteogenesis imperfecta, osteomyelitis and certain endocrine imbalances.

Osteoporosis produces a tendency to fracture of the neck of femur, especially in the elderly female. The bone is not mineral-deficient, as in the case of osteomalacia. Treatment of generalized osteoporosis is directed at maintaining weightbearing mobility and the use of oestrogens, calcium and vitamin D.

The general aims of treatment for a fracture are to:

- relieve pain;
- reduce the fracture to a good anatomical position;
- immobilize the fracture to promote healing;
- restore function.

Fractures of the femoral shaft

Treatment depends mainly on the age of the patient. Conservative treatment is by traction, using a Thomas's splint, for three months. Alternatively, a cast-brace or plaster cylinder may be fitted after partial union of the fracture at eight weeks. Internal fixation of a fractured femoral shaft involves the use of an intramedullary nail. This has the advantage of allowing weightbearing within one to two weeks and is therefore preferable for the older patient.

Fractures of the hip

Fracture of the neck of femur at the subcapital site is the most common in the elderly patient. In approximately 5% of these cases, the two fragments are impacted with slight abduction of the femur. This fracture is stable and may be fixed by various means, including Garden screws, a nail and plate or with a compression screw and plate (Figures 3.4, 3.5 and 3.6).

Intertrochanteric fractures of the hip are treated by compression screw or nail and plate. Subtrochanteric fractures are fixed by intramedullary rod or compression screw and long plate.

In the other 95% of cases of fractured neck of femur, the bone ends are displaced, usually with the shaft rotated and displaced upwards due to the pull of the thigh muscles. The leg is rotated laterally, there is limb shortening and severe pain on movement. Treatment is by internal fixation to avoid the complications arising from prolonged bedrest in the elderly, i.e. hypostatic pneumonia, osteoporosis, muscle wasting, pressure sores and urinary tract infections. The most probable surgical procedures are:

- compression screw and plate. The dynamic hip screw is a variation of this;
- excision of the femoral head, followed by hemi-arthroplasty;
- total hip replacement.

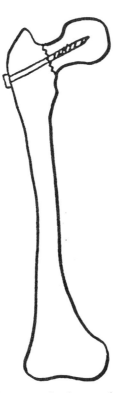

Figure 3.4 Garden screw for fractured neck of femur

Reasons for more radical surgery include:

1. The blood supply to the head and neck of the femur may be severely disrupted by the fracture, leading to avascular necrosis and collapse of the head and neck of femur later.
2. Approximately one third of these fractures fail to unite or are slow to do so. If this occurs, the neck of the femur is gradually absorbed, the head of femur and trochanter come closer together, the fixation loosens and the bone fragments displace.
3. Secondary osteo-arthritis often follows fractured neck of femur.

Hemi-arthroplasty

The advantage of replacement of the femoral head is the rapid relief of pain and return to mobility. The Thompson hemi-arthroplasty and the Austin-Moore prosthesis are commonly used (Figure 3.7).

The cause of pathological fracture of the neck of femur must be sought and treated. It may be due to osteomyelitis, osteomalacia, tumour, following radia-

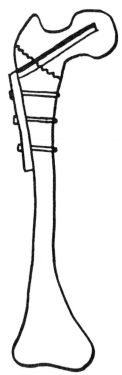

Figure 3.5 Nail and plate fixation for intertrochanteric feature of femur

tion, Paget's disease and some forms of rickets. These fractures may not unite if the bone is infected or if there is a malignant tumour.

The patient is up mobilizing a few days after surgery. The physiotherapist teaches static quadriceps exercises. Muscle power must be restored early to prevent atrophy and joint stiffness. Every part of the body should be exercised as much as possible to maintain physical strength and stimulate the circulation, which promotes healing.

The aims of occupational therapy are:

- to keep the patient as active and mobile as possible, to promote healing;
- to enable the patient to be independent in ADL;
- to encourage a gradual return to full activity.

To this end the patient should be encouraged to dress in day clothes and look after his personal needs, given the necessary tools. These tools will be similar to those required following total hip replacement and assessment should broadly follow the same lines. The patient who has had hemi-arthroplasty should take the same precautions as for total hip replacement. The pinned and plated femur will be somewhat stiff, but there is no danger of dislocation.

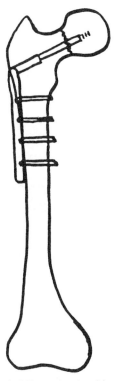

Figure 3.6 Compression hip screw

AMBULATION TRAINING

Although this is the responsibility of the physiotherapist, ambulation is all-important in the rehabilitation of patients following hip surgery and the occupational therapist reinforces the teaching of the physiotherapist when she is retraining the patient in daily living activities.

When the patient is non-weightbearing he uses crutches. If axillary crutches are used, the patient should push down onto the handgrips with his hands and the crutch pads should be two fingers' width from the axillae. The crutch tips are placed six to eight inches either side of the patient's feet and the handgrips adjusted so that the elbows are in 15° of flexion.

If the patient is non-weightbearing, the three point gait is used. The crutches are moved forward together, then the good leg swung forward to a point either just ahead of or just behind the crutches, which is a more stable position than with the foot in line with the crutches.

At home, the patient may have to negotiate stairs. Unless the physiotherapist is present, the occupational therapist must be certain of the technique for stair

49

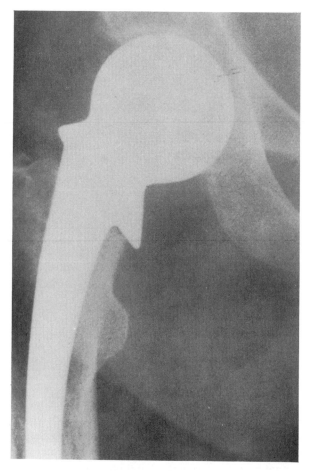

Figure 3.7 Austin-Moore prosthesis for fractured neck of femur

management with crutches. It is important that a sturdy handrail is in situ before stairs are attempted. The two crutches are held in one hand, one in position for support, the second held at right angles to it. Alternatively, the second crutch may be left downstairs and a third crutch kept upstairs. The good leg goes up first followed by the crutch, and when descending stairs, the crutch is put on the lower step first followed by the good leg.

For partial weightbearing, axillary or elbow crutches may be used. The bad leg and both crutches are brought forward together, the amount of weight borne depending on the amount of pressure the patient puts through the crutches. This method is used for 'toe-touching' or minimal weightbearing.

The two point gait is the usual method for partial weightbearing. One crutch and the opposite foot are brought forward together, then the opposite crutch and the second foot brought forward.

For full weightbearing the four point gait is used, with one stick being put forward, followed by the opposite leg, then the second stick put forward, then the second foot. This is the usual method of ambulation taught to patients being discharged home on two sticks.

Although hip patients have normally progressed to sticks before discharge from hospital, it may be advisable for a walking frame to be provided for a short time after discharge for the patient who has to get up to use the toilet in the night.

REFERENCES

Hughes, S. (1989) *A New Short Textbook of Orthopaedics and Traumatology*, Edward Arnold, London.

FURTHER READING

Beary III, J.F. *et al.* (1987) *Manual of Rheumatology and Outpatient Orthopaedic Disorders*, 2nd edn, Little Brown Medical, London.

Browne, P.S.H. (1985) *Basic Facts in Orthopaedics*, 2nd edn, Blackwell Scientific Publications, Oxford.

Calvert, P.T., August, A.C., Albert, J.S., Kemp, H.B. and Catterall A. (1987) The Chiari pelvic osteotomy, *Journal of Bone and Joint Surgery*, **69-B**, no. 4, 551–5.

Crenshaw, A.H. (ed.) (1987) *Campbell's Operative Procedures Vol. 4*, Mosby, St Louis.

Davies, M. (1988) Sexual problems and physical disability, in C.J. Goodwill and M.A. Chamberlain (eds.) *Rehabilitation of the Physically Disabled Adult*, Croom Helm /Sheridan Medical, London.

Fisher, J. and Jackson, M. (1988) Walking aids, in C.J. Goodwill and M.A. Chamberlain (eds.) *Rehabilitation of the Physically Disabled Adult*, Croom Helm /Sheridan Medical, London.

Hardinge, K. (1983) *Hip Replacement: The facts*, Oxford University Press, Oxford.

Hogh, J. and MacNicol, M.F. (1987) The Chiari pelvic osteotomy, *Journal of Bone and Joint Surgery*, **69-B**, no. 3, 363–73.

Osterkamp, J.O., Caillouette, J.T. and Hoffer, M.M. (1988) Chiari osteotomy in cerebral palsy, *Journal of Paediatric Orthopaedics*, **8**, no. 3, 274–7.

Pedretti, L.W. (1981) *Occupational Therapy Practice Skills for Physical Dysfunction*, Mosby, St Louis.

Trombly, C. (1983) *Occupational Therapy for Physical Dysfunction*, 2nd edn, Williams and Wilkins, Baltimore.

Zlatic, M. *et al.* (1988) Late results of Chiari's pelvic osteotomy, *International Orthopaedics*, **12,** 149–54.

4

Knee surgery

While occupational therapists in medical rehabilitation centres carry out heavy workshop activities with patients following some knee surgery, many patients undergoing elective surgery for knee conditions remain in hospital for a very short time and there may be insufficient incapacity to merit occupational therapy intervention. Occupational therapy input is necessary for rheumatoid arthritis affecting the knee joint (see Chapter 1 for pathology, etc.) and also for osteo-arthritis of the knee.

OSTEO-ARTHRITIS OF THE KNEE

The actual disease process as it affects the joint is as described for osteo-arthritis of the hip. It is mainly the elderly who are affected and the condition is aggravated by obesity. If the medial compartment of the knee is affected, genu varum (bow leg) results, and if the lateral compartment is affected, it causes genu valgum (knock knee). Secondary osteo-arthritis may result from an old injury or from recurrent dislocation of the patella.

Arthritic knees restrict the patient's mobility when walking, negotiating stairs, rising from chairs and bending to tie shoelaces or cut toenails. Because of the pain, the patient spends more time in his chair, resulting in increased immobility due to wasting of the quadriceps muscles in particular and stiffening of the joint, sometimes to the point of developing a fixed flexion deformity. If this occurs the patient is still further incapacitated. Treatment is by physiotherapy to strengthen the quadriceps muscles and stretch out flexion contracture. Serial splinting may be required to achieve the latter. The patient should rest with the knee in extension. Anti-inflammatory drugs are prescribed and an injection of hydrocortisone directly into the joint affords pain relief.

If the patient is obese his weight should be reduced. Walking aids are provided to reduce the weight being put through the joints. Occupational therapy intervention is directed at provision of tools to maintain independence and to relieve the pain of struggling with difficult daily activities. Tools for living required may include:

- high seat chair and legrest;
- bedraising devices;
- raised toilet seat and/or toilet frame, or handrail on wall;
- bathing aids;
- second stair-rail;
- grabrails by big access steps;
- long shoehorn;
- sock/stocking or tights aids;
- elastic shoelaces.

If the patient is unable to have knee surgery for health reasons, he may deteriorate to the point of a wheelchair existence. Knee arthroplasty offers pain relief and restores mobility.

TOTAL KNEE REPLACEMENT

The knee is a more difficult joint for successful replacement than the hip as its structure is more complex. There are two separate articulations within the one joint, i.e. the patello-femoral and the tibio-femoral joints. The tibio-femoral is a modified hinge joint, flexion and extension being the main movements, but some rotation with the knee in flexion and very slight passive abduction and adduction take place. Strong ligaments and tendons provide stability. The knee works in conjunction with the hip and ankle joints in supporting the body weight when standing erect. It is therefore a major stabilizing joint and also a major mobilizing joint, enabling walking, sitting, kneeling, squatting and kicking. The medial compartment of the tibio-femoral joint and the patello-femoral joint are most commonly affected by arthritis and, at later stages, all three compartments are destroyed.

Although a knee replacement may be performed with confidence on the older, less active patient, the results are on the whole somewhat less satisfactory than with hip replacement.

There are varying types of prosthesis, including the surface replacement, the hinge, the unicompartmental, the patello-femoral and the rotating hinge replacement. The hinge type prosthesis (e.g. the Stanmore total knee replacement) produces a simple flexion and extension movement, suitable when there is considerable joint destruction in the more infirm patient. This type of prosthesis is prone to loosening in an active patient.

With the surface type of prosthesis (e.g. the Kinematic total knee replacement, Figure 4.1), each articular surface is properly shaped and a metal femoral component is cemented in place over the femoral condyles and a polyethylene component attached to the tibia. An optional extra is a polyethylene component for the articular surface of the patella. This prosthesis more nearly imitates the

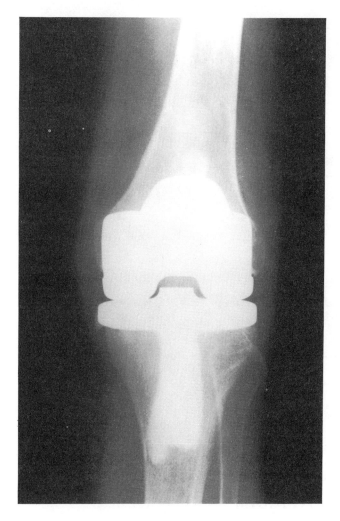

Figure 4.1 Total knee replacement, Kinematic type (a) anterio-posterior

natural knee joint, but must be aligned very carefully and depends on strong ligaments for stability.

The rotating hinge prosthesis, as its name suggests, allows flexion, extension and rotation and the link prosthesis is an example of this type.

The successful total knee replacement produces a stable, painfree knee with at least 90° of flexion.

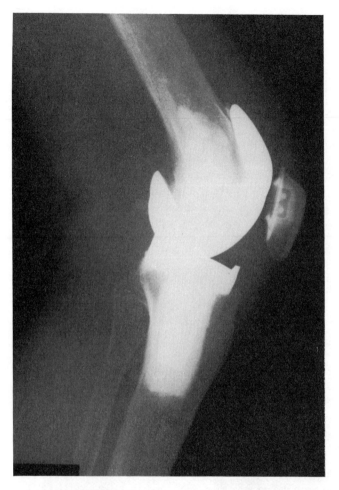

Figure 4.1 Total knee replacement, (b) lateral view

REVISION OF TOTAL KNEE REPLACEMENT

The most common reasons for revision of knee replacement are loosening and deep infection, although loosening of the newer implants is less common. Other reasons include patellar problems such as subluxation, dislocation and fractures. Poor axial alignment may lead to stress at the bone–cement interface, causing loosening. The failure rate of the older hinged prosthesis is high, but the less constrained prosthesis causes less stress at the interface.

There are many factors to be considered when revision is to be undertaken: the reason for failure of the primary, possible infection, deficient bone stock and/or supporting soft tissues, balancing of the collateral ligaments, ease of removal of the old implant and the patient's motivation for rehabilitation.

Surgeons have their own preferences for the type of implant they employ for revision surgery. The greater the bone loss and instability, the more need there is for a more constrained type of prosthesis. A condylar prosthesis is suitable only when bone stock and collateral ligaments are good. An intramedullary stem may provide better fixation.

Removal of the old implant is time-consuming and often difficult, especially with a porous coated implant, and significant bone loss may result. Where there is infection every particle of old cement must be removed. If the bone stock is satisfactory, insertion of the new prosthesis is as for the primary, in one or two stages, as for revision surgery of the hip. Antibiotic-loaded acrylic cement is commonly used in the revision of infected knee implants. Bone grafts and allografts are used to make up deficient bone stock. When bone stock is very poor, custom-made endoprosthetic replacements may be used.

After revision of total knee replacement, mobilization is more difficult and the post-operative programme is individualized. Results are generally less good than for primary arthroplasty. There is sometimes extension lag. Surgery is considered successful if the patient has little or no pain, if he can flex the knee to 90° and if the joint is stable. A survey has demonstrated that the success rate for revised knee replacements declines gradually for each subsequent revision (Rand and Bryan, 1988). In patients with rheumatoid arthritis, the survival rate of the prosthesis is better than for those with osteo-arthritis, probably because the patient with rheumatoid disease is less active.

Precautions following revision include avoidance of lifting more than 30 lbs (13.5 kg) weight, no kneeling and no sudden change in direction, acceleration or deceleration.

OSTEOTOMY

If the knee joint is painful and deformed but still reasonably mobile, tibial osteotomy may be performed. This operation is dependent on the joint surfaces being relatively intact. It is a solution to the genu varum deformity. A wedge of bone is removed from the lateral aspect of the tibia just below the knee joint. The bone is then re-aligned in the correct position, so that the weight is transferred directly down the leg. Alternatively, a dome upper tibial osteotomy can be performed (Figure 4.2). Recovery is slow and the operation is used more for younger patients. Valgus deformity of the knee is better treated with a supracondylar medial wedge osteotomy.

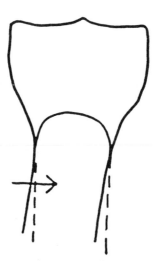

Figure 4.2 Dome tibial osteotomy

ARTHRODESIS

The most likely candidate for knee arthrodesis is the patient with severe rheumatoid arthritis or chronic infection of the knee. While this surgery relieves pain, it causes another disability and may be performed on one knee only. The articulating surfaces of the tibio-femoral joint are excised and the two bones firmly fixed together by means of a long Kuntscher nail, or by external fixation using compression clamps. The knee then becomes stable but because it is now stiff, the patient's leg projects awkwardly when sitting so that it is difficult to accommodate when using public transport, when getting in and out of many types of car, and creates problems when negotiating stairs.

PATELLECTOMY

This is occasionally performed on patients with arthritis affecting only the patello-femoral joint, or for chondromalacia of the patella. The latter condition may be caused by trauma or recurrent dislocation of the patella, distorting the articular cartilage. This produces pain, possible effusion into the joint, and allows the knee to give way.

DEBRIDEMENT

Loose pieces of bone and cartilage sometimes separate from the bone ends and float about inside the joint, causing pain and loss of function. The loose particles are removed and the irregular surfaces trimmed. The outcome is variable and the long term effects of doubtful value. Knee replacement at a later date is likely.

OCCUPATIONAL THERAPY

Patients recovering from total knee replacement are required to achieve 90° of knee flexion before discharge. If the knee flexion is not satisfactory after two weeks, manipulation under anaesthetic may be carried out. A continuous passive motion (CPM) machine which continually flexes and extends the knee is used for some part of each day. Because of the good range of knee flexion achieved before discharge, patients are on the whole not in need of any tools for living, provided the contralateral knee is reasonably sound. Many patients develop good hip flexion to compensate for the knee restriction pre-operatively, so dressing the lower half is usually no problem.

However, if bilateral knee replacement is carried out simultaneously, if the other knee is arthritic or if the patient suffers from rheumatoid arthritis, occupational therapy intervention is necessary. Occupational therapy aims and objectives are similar to those for hip replacement (see p. 33). Equipment which may be required includes:

- raised toilet seat and/or toilet frame or handrails on wall;
- high seat chair;
- bedraising devices;
- bath board and possibly bath seat.

If the hip joints are also arthritic, the patient needs tools for living as previously described for arthritic hips but it is usual for the hip joints to be replaced first.

If the patient has rheumatoid arthritis, he needs a full occupational therapy assessment as described in Chapter 1, mainly because his upper limbs should not be stressed in an attempt to protect the new knees when rising from the sitting position. The same considerations apply to patients who have had patellectomy or tibial osteotomy.

The patient with an arthrodesed knee needs occupational therapy intervention. Depending on the method of fixation, he will be discharged home to await healing either in a plaster cylinder from groin to ankle, or with compression rods still in situ. Occupational therapy aims are similar to those for hip arthrodesis. If in a cylinder plaster, the patient may need:

- raised toilet seat with a dip side to accommodate the plaster, and possibly a toilet frame;
- high seat chair and legrest;
- sock gutter to put on short sock to keep foot warm;
- long shoehorn and elastic shoelaces;
- long-handled sponge to reach the foot.

Mounting and descending stairs must be done in the child's manner already described.

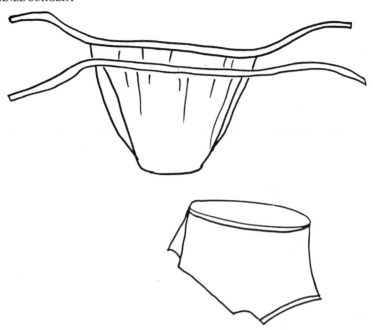

Figure 4.3 Pants adaptations for use with external fixation operations

If the patient is discharged wearing the apparatus for external fixation, he needs the above equipment plus a bed cradle to protect the sheets from the metalwork. He will appreciate advice on wrapping old sheeting or similar around the ends of the metal bars to protect the lower sheet. Looselegged pants are needed over a cylinder plaster. Over external fixation, loose pants are needed, possibly with the side seam opened up and a temporary gusset inserted. Sidefastening underpants can be substituted, similar to baby waterproof pants, obtainable from specialist suppliers (address in appendix). Alternatively a garment may be made up as illustrated and tied over the hips (Figure 4.3).

Once the knee has arthrodesed, the patient needs the listed equipment plus bathing aids permanently. A bath board or a stool at least as high as the side of the bath enables the patient to raise the leg over the side of the bath. If he drives a British car, he will have difficulty bringing his right leg into the car, if that is the one which is arthrodesed. He must be given the necessary information in case he needs adaptations to his car. He will get used to sitting at the end of a row of seats in places of entertainment and by the gangway on the appropriate side if travelling by public transport.

The success of coping after this operation depends on the condition of the opposite knee and on the strength of the patient's arms. Clearly, only one knee can be arthrodesed, so the other knee must be either unaffected or should be assessed as suitable for replacement. If the latter, a stair lift may be necessary to prevent additional stress on the knee replacement.

LIMB LENGTH DISCREPANCY

The usual causes of this condition are:

1. True shortening due to:
   - congenital or developmental abnormality;
   - growth arrest at the epiphysis due to trauma or infection;
   - overgrowth caused by a healing fracture or osteotomy.
2. Apparent shortening, due to hip dislocation or pelvic obliquity.

Surgical correction of this condition depends on the accurate calculation of bone growth, based on the normal growth at specific skeletal ages. The distal femoral epiphysis contributes 37% to total growth of the leg, while the proximal tibial epiphysis contributes 28%. The relative size of the individual is taken into account and the timing of surgery is crucial.

Surgical methods of femoral shortening are only applicable for differences of less than 5 cm and obviously result in loss of height. In theory, limb lengthening is preferable. The three principal methods are the Wagner mid-diaphyseal osteotomy and the DeBastiani and Ilizarov methods of callotasis (callus distraction).

In the Wagner method, when the required distraction gap is achieved it is packed with cancellous bone graft and internally fixed. When the graft is solid the fixation is removed and replaced with a semi-flexible tubular plate, which is later removed when the medullary canal and cortex formation have become normal. The patient is partially weightbearing throughout.

The DeBastiani technique involves proximal submetaphyseal corticotomy, with distraction at 1 mm daily commenced 10–14 days later, using a dynamic axial fixator. This fixator is locked rigid when the required distraction is achieved and when bone consolidation has occurred, the fixator screw is released and dynamic axial loading commenced until cortex formation has become normal.

The Ilizarov method involves proximal corticotomy of the tibia, close to the metaphysis. The Ilizarov frame is a device in which wires pass through bone and soft tissue from one side of the limb to another, at multiple levels and in several planes, in order to achieve stability (Figure 4.4). Cyclic axial dynamization occurs which stimulates bone regeneration. Distraction is commenced at 10–14 days post-operatively and proceeds at the rate of 1 mm per day. The frame is removed when the medullary canal and cortex formation have become normal, the regenerated bone is clinically stable and the patient feels the limb firm beneath his weight (Tachdjian, 1990).

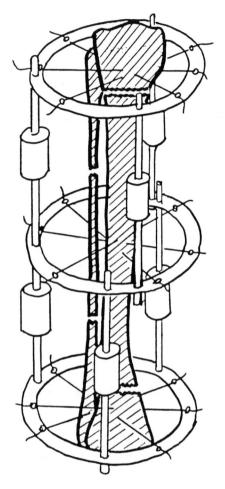

Figure 4.4 Ilizarov frame for leg lengthening surgery

Indications for the Ilizarov method of distraction osteogenesis are limb length discrepancy of more than 5 cm and functional impairment. Contra-indications are joint instability and poor bone stock. The patient must be well motivated and cooperate with the treatment.

Physiotherapy is directed at maintaining and increasing the range of movement of the joints above and below the site of surgery, plus increasing muscle power.

Occupational therapy intervention is mainly aimed at provision of a suitable wheelchair for outdoor use. If the femur is lengthened, additional width in the wheelchair seat is necessary to accommodate the fixator. If the lower leg is lengthened, an elevating legrest is needed. The home will need provision of ramps to facilitate access. Provision of other tools for living is as for external fixation of the arthrodesed knee (see p.59).

REFERENCES

Rand, J.A. and Bryan, R.S. (1988) Results of revision total knee arthroplasties using condylar prostheses, *Journal of Bone and Joint Surgery*, **70-A**, no. 5, 738–44.

Tachdjian, M.O. (1990) *Paediatric Orthopaedics Vol. 4*, W.B. Saunders, Philadelphia.

FURTHER READING

Browne, P.S.H. (1985) *Basic Facts in Orthopaedics*, 2nd edn, Blackwell Scientific Publications, Oxford.

Hanssen, A.D. and Rand, J.A. (1988) A comparison of primary and revision total knee arthroplasty using the Kinematic stabilizer prosthesis, *Journal of Bone and Joint Surgery*, **70-A**, no. 4, 491–8.

Hardinge, K. (1983) *Hip Replacement: The facts*, Oxford University Press, Oxford.

Hughes S. (1989) *A New Short Textbook of Orthopaedics and Traumatology*, Edward Arnold, London.

Insall, J.N. (1986) *Revision of Total Knee Arthroplasty*, Instructional Course Lectures, American Academy of Orthopaedic Surgeons, Chicago.

Kaufer, H. and Matthews, L.S. (1986) *Revision of Total Knee Arthroplasty: Indications and contra-indications*, Instructional Course Lectures, American Academy of Orthopaedic Surgeons, Chicago.

Norkin, C. and Levangie, P. (1989) *Joint Structure and Function : A comprehensive analysis,* F.A. Davis, Philadelphia.

Rand, J.A., Peterson, L.F.A., Bryan, R.S. and Ilstrup, D.M. (1986) *Revision of Total Knee Arthroplasty*, Instructional Course Lectures, American Academy of Orthopaedic Surgeons, Chicago.

5

Back pain

The spine supports the whole body and is involved in almost every movement we make. A series of curves provides resilience and absorbs shock as we walk. There is an extensive ligamentous system to the spine which, with the vertebral muscles, supports the spinal column. Nerve roots are situated close to the spinal structures and may become trapped or subjected to pressure, particularly in the lumbar spine where the stresses are greatest at L4–L5 and L5–S1 levels.

In Britain, approximately 33,000,000 working days are lost each year through back complaints (Tanner, 1987). The highest incidence is in the middle years, when the most stress is put on the spine. Causes of low back pain include:

* heavy manual work;
* incorrect lifting techniques;
* poor posture;
* obesity;
* poor working conditions: poorly designed furniture, inaccessible controls, restricted space, etc.;
* long distance driving;
* pregnancy, lifting and carrying children;
* physically less fit as age advances;
* sports undertaken by older age group, e.g. bowls and golf, which involve bending and twisting.

Most low back pain is the result of mechanical problems, due to poor body mechanics, structural abnormality or defective vertebrae. A smaller percentage of back pain is caused by inflammation, infection or spinal tumours. In low back pain resulting from internal organic problems such as kidney or uterine disorders, the pain is unaffected by mobility.

Back pain is manifested in many ways and the treatment and outcome are variable.

MECHANICAL PROBLEMS

The annulus fibrosus, or outer layer of the intervertebral discs, is composed of fibrous cartilage. The nucleus pulposus, or inner part, is flexible and gel-like.

The discs act as shock absorbers between the vertebrae. They do not 'slip' but they can prolapse due to sudden heavy work when an individual is out of condition, e.g. digging the garden in spring. Heavy lifting, especially when combined with rotation of the spine, may cause the outer layer of cartilage to rupture, allowing the nucleus to protrude and press on the posterior longitudinal ligament, causing back pain. If the disc presses on the nerve root it will cause pain to travel down the leg, possibly with pins and needles or numbness in the area supplied by that nerve. The straight leg raise is often reduced (normal flexion is 70 – 90°) and this, with signs of nerve root compression, is the routine diagnostic test for the condition.

Facet joint strain is caused by the vertebrae being misaligned due to slack ligaments or to a twisting or jolting injury. Pain may radiate to the thighs or buttocks but there is no sharp pain or numbness down the leg.

After the age of 30 years, the intervertebral discs begin to dry out, resulting in space narrowing and degeneration by the age of 60. This disc degeneration may cause problems with the facet joints as they are deformed. This causes low back pain when standing and inability to lie prone. In the early stages, attention to posture and exercises will be helpful. Spondylosis, or degenerative arthritis, is a sequel of disc degeneration. Osteophytes may grow on the intervertebral joints and may cause narrowing of the spinal canal, resulting in trapped nerves and compressed blood vessels. The condition is known as spinal canal stenosis and the symptoms are pins and needles, numbness, cramps and pains in the legs on walking. The symptoms are relieved by sitting down or bending forwards, which widens the spinal canal. Patients with this complaint may be able to cycle and walk upstairs in comfort, in spite of severe limitation in walking distance.

Sacro-iliac joint pain is commonly caused by pregnancy and is a nagging ache, aggravated by bending and twisting.

Ligament injuries heal slowly and sometimes incompletely, causing chronic low back pain. The ligaments tend to harden in old age so the spine stiffens and stabilizes.

Spondylolysis is a small crack across the neural arch. It may be congenital or due to a fall onto the bottom, or occur as a stress fracture in sports people.

Spondylolisthesis may develop as a sequel to spondylolysis. Part of the vertebra may fracture and displace, causing deformity. Treatment is by decompression or spinal fusion.

Scoliosis is a lateral spinal curve, occurring in childhood or adolescence. Since it causes deformity and early degeneration, surgery is usually required.

Fractures of the vertebrae are usually due to falls, road traffic accidents or sports injuries. There is a possibility of spinal cord damage, in which case the patient is usually transferred to the nearest spinal injuries centre. It is not within the scope of this book to cover this subject. The condition which is more likely to be met on the orthopaedic ward is the crush fracture of the vertebra, which occurs in the osteoporotic spine. The vertebra becomes wedge-shaped and the deformity tends to remain as kyphosis or scoliosis. Treatment is by rest and analgesics. Keeping elderly people physically active helps to prevent these fractures because stress on bone encourages the osteoblasts to lay down new bone cells.

Non-specific back pain has various causes, possibly the most common being poor posture. There are differing manifestations of poor posture, but that most likely to cause low back pain is the stance with exaggerated pelvic tilt and slack abdominal muscles. The condition is aggravated by obesity and wearing high-heeled shoes. Poor sitting posture in soft chairs with inadequate lumbar support causes stretched ligaments in the lumbar area.

Sports people, gymnasts and dancers are prone to non-specific back pain. Their joints tend to be hypermobile, leading to premature 'wear and tear'.

In myofascial dysfunction, taut 'knots' occur in the muscle, causing pain which is aggravated by exercise. An example is the muscle spasm in the trapezium muscle over the upper scapula, causing referred pain into the neck and base of the skull. Such cases often respond to local injection of novocaine.

Psychological pressure causes tension in the back muscles, producing pain. Frequently patients presenting with this kind of pain with no clear physical cause are dismissed as attempting to opt out of difficult situations. This is possible but the patient should be assessed very carefully, since his pain may be genuine and he needs help, be it physical or psychological.

NON-MECHANICAL PROBLEMS

The following conditions produce back pain as a result of inflammation or disease.

Tuberculosis of the spine is the most common infection, occurring mainly in the Asian community. Back pain develops insidiously and is not relieved by rest. The systemic symptoms of tuberculosis are present: pyrexia, night sweats, weight loss and debility. Treatment is by antibiotics and excision of the diseased bone, followed by spinal fusion with bone grafting.

Osteomyelitis is an infection of a vertebral body, which may eventually collapse, with probable neurological complications. A local abscess may occur as a further complication. The precise cause must be identified and specific antibiotics prescribed. A plaster cast is applied to prevent spinal deformity and the area usually fuses in three to six months.

Osteomalacia is a disease similar in effect to osteoporosis. The bones weaken, small crush fractures of the vertebrae and consequent stoop develop and there is loss of weight. Vegan Asians are prone to it due to dietary deficiency. Treatment is by a few days rest, plus administration of calcium and vitamin D, hormone replacement therapy and sodium fluoride.

Paget's disease is the excessive formation of dense bone with areas of rarefaction, therefore a tendency towards pathological fracture. Back pain may be due also to spinal canal stenosis. Treatment is either by injection of calcitonin which lowers the blood calcium and makes it available to the bones, or by diphosphonates.

Arachnoiditis is inflammation of the nerve sheaths in the spinal canal, which can no longer glide smoothly through the intervertebral foramina. It may be the result of an earlier injury or due to a now discontinued form of spinal investigation. Pain is persistent, with possible feelings of heat or tingling in the limbs. It is unrelated to movement but may be relieved by trunk extension. It is treated mainly by analgesics as there is a high recurrence rate after surgery.

Ankylosing spondylitis causes back pain of non-mechanical nature (see Chapter 1).

Bone tumours may be primary or, more usually, metastatic (see Chapter 10). If the tumour is intraspinal, pain will be accompanied by progressive neurological signs.

DIAGNOSTIC TESTS

The surgeon will observe the patient's movements and will test for extension and for forward and lateral flexion of the spine, nerve root involvement, sensation and power. He will check for leg length discrepancy and rotation of the hips to exclude them as the cause of pain. The patient will be asked to describe his pain, its severity, how it may be triggered, whether it occurs at rest, how often it occurs, etc. A nerve pain is sharp and precise in location, while pain from inflamed soft tissues is dull and vague in location.

Radiographs demonstrate some abnormalities, such as increased lumbar lordosis, scoliosis, narrowed disc space, osteo-arthritis, spondylolisthesis and facet joint asymmetry. Many spinal abnormalities do not show up and specific tests may be necessary.

For radiculogram, a special dye injected into the vertebral canal occupies the space behind the vertebral bodies and the discs, so that any protrusion of the disc blocks the flow of dye. The lesion will then appear on X-ray.

Discogram involves a radio-opaque fluid being injected under anaesthetic directly into the intervertebral disc, using X-ray to guide the needle. This precisely identifies a disc problem.

Computerized axial tomography (CAT) scan reveals soft tissue abnormality as well as bone. A beam of X-rays is passed through the body and records a transmitted signal on the other side, this information being processed by computer. In this way, pictures of slices across the patient's body enable more accurate diagnosis.

Magnetic resonance imaging (MRI) is a development from the CAT scan, giving a very finely detailed picture. As X-rays are not used, it is thought to be without risk and the procedure is entirely painless.

When a bone scan is performed, a solution containing a minute amount of radio-active material is injected into a vein and is taken up by the bones, any hyperactive areas showing up as 'hot spots'. These areas may be due to infection, healing fracture or a tumour. The scan provides an early and very accurate diagnosis. There is a wait of two to three hours between injection and scan. There are no side effects.

NON-SURGICAL MANAGEMENT OF BACK PAIN

The aims of treatment are to:

- alleviate pain;
- restore function/mobility;
- avoid residual disability;
- prevent recurrence;
- prevent development of chronic back pain.

The basic treatments are:

1. Bedrest. Inflamed tissues are rested and gravity eliminated. A firm mattress and one pillow only is allowed and the treatment continued for up to three weeks.
2. Analgesics and, if indicated, non-steroid anti-inflammatory drugs (NSAIDs).
3. Pelvic traction. The lower end of the bed is raised and the traction pulls upwards on the pelvis, decreasing the lordosis, opening up the foramina, minimizing any annular bulging and overcoming spasm of the erector spinae muscles.
4. Immobilization in a corset. This helps to relieve muscle spasm and improve posture by decreasing the lumbar lordosis and supporting the abdominal muscles. It is a possible substitute for bedrest in milder cases.
5. Manipulation. There must be a full medical assessment before manipulation, since it is of no benefit in the treatment of a prolapsed disc and can be disastrous where disease is present. A chiropractor aims to reposition specific vertebrae with thrusting techniques. The osteopath uses rhythmic stretching of ligaments around the offending joint(s) to restore range of movement.

Mobilization phase

The aims of exercise are to:

1. restore normal range of movement;
2. improve the power of the spinal and abdominal muscles, thereby reducing stress on bones and joints;
3. improve posture to prevent recurrence.

Mobilization should be gradual after complete bedrest. Extremes of movement and any stretching of an irritable nerve must be avoided. The physiotherapist will teach specific exercises, depending on the site and cause of the pain. Pelvic tilting and spinal extension exercises are commonly taught.

Patients frequently ask what type of exercise they may safely undertake. When walking, the arms should be free to swing, which produces a few degrees of rotation with weightbearing which improves the strength of the annular fibres of the discs. Swimming provides excellent exercise, apart from breast stroke if the swimmer holds his head clear of the water. Cycling is good, provided upright handlebars are used and a spongy saddle to absorb shock.

Posture

When standing correctly, a plumbline should pass in front of the ear, through the shoulder, just behind the lumbar curve, through the hip joint and just in front of the knee and ankle. Slight variations may occur, depending on the individual's body shape. If posture is correct, balance is maintained using minimal energy. Conversely, poor posture results in imbalance, fatigue and possible pain.

Two concepts of posture exist, one emphasizing the importance of decreasing the pelvic tilt, the other advocating maintaining the lumbar lordosis at all times. Cailliet (1988) believes both have their merits depending on the individual patient.

Posture is influenced by heredity, culture, occupation, mechanical abnormalities and habits formed early in life, which become deep-seated in neuromuscular proprioception. Posture modification requires time and commitment and monitoring by a professional person.

Pedretti (1981) lists the correct postures for proper body mechanics as follows:

1. Sitting: use a lumbar support in the chair, or a footstool. Get up and move around every 45 minutes (this is an arbitrary figure).
2. Lying: on the back, use a pillow under the knees. On the side, use a pillow between the legs.
3. Lifting: keep feet apart, bend knees, tighten abdominal muscles, avoid twisting, retain lumbar lordosis, hold object close.
4. Carrying: as for lifting and hold object at waist level.
5. Reaching: if above the shoulders, use steps.
6. Pushing: in preference to pulling. Push with legs or entire body weight to initiate movement.
7. Pulling: avoid if possible. If it must be done, retain the lumbar lordosis, bend knees, keep feet well apart, use body weight to pull, not back muscles.
8. Mounting stairs: walk on the front part of the foot.

The Back School

The Back School concept is directed at the patient with persistent back pain to enable him to take some control of his own treatment (Cailliet, 1988). Its aims are:

- to enable the patient to be independent in ADL;
- to encourage a positive attitude and maintain a normal lifestyle;
- to improve the condition of the tissues needed for proper function;
- to assist recovery and prevent recurrence of pain.

The objectives are to enable the patient, following instruction and practice:

- to understand the basic anatomy and physiology of his back;
- to strengthen and maintain in good trim the musculature of his spine and abdomen, by regular performance of specific exercises;
- to be aware of, and avoid, harmful positions and activities;
- to perform all necessary ADL tasks, with the aid of any tools deemed necessary.

The Back School may be run by the physiotherapist or the occupational therapist, or both together. Typically, the programme is covered in four to six sessions over a period of two weeks or more. This programme consists of:

1. explanation of the basic anatomy and physiology of the spine;
2. instruction in body mechanics, i.e. use of the spine with the least amount of stress;
3. instruction of exercises to build up tolerance and endurance, improve posture and, in the upper limbs, to aid lifting and carrying. patients are warned to stop an exercise if it causes pain;
4. advice on how to approach all aspects of daily living activity, to put the least stress on the spine;
5. instruction in energy conservation;
6. advice on stress management and instruction in simple relaxation techniques.

If this Back School concept was incorporated into the orientation programme when employees started a new job, the employers could take steps to minimize the risk of injury by identifying the potentially damaging tasks and educating the employees accordingly. The scheme would be of mutual benefit to employer and employee.

Physiotherapy for persistent back pain

In addition to the exercises and postural training, the physiotherapist may use any of the following in the treatment of back pain:

- hydrotherapy;
- massage;
- ice packs;
- superficial heat, especially before exercise or manipulation;
- ultrasound, especially for sports injuries;
- short wave diathermy (a high frequency wave which promotes tissue healing);
- interferential (a low frequency wave which reduces inflammation and temporarily relieves pain);
- transcutaneous electrical nerve stimulation (TENS).

This last is based on the 'gate' control theory of pain perception which is discussed in Chapter 11.

THE ANAESTHETIST'S ARMOURY

When back pain has failed to respond to the foregoing forms of non-surgical treatment, the anaesthetist has at his disposal the following methods of pain relief:

1. Lumbar epidural injection. This consists of a local anaesthetic and soluble steroid injected into the epidural space, used in the treatment of sciatic pain. A second or third injection may be necessary at weekly intervals. For more intractable problems, an indwelling catheter may be employed, topped up as necessary.
2. Nerve root block injection. This is used only after all other treatment has failed. Local anaesthetic and steroid are injected into the specific nerve root.
3. Facet joint injections. The local anaesthetic and steroid are injected directly into the damaged facet joint.

Other techniques are available but these three are most widely used.

OCCUPATIONAL THERAPY ASSESSMENT

The occupational therapist must first acquaint herself with the patient's medical history. At the initial interview she must explain her role regarding his treatment. She should then ask about his home situation; whether he lives alone, in what type of accommodation, what support is available, what special responsibilities he has, etc. If he is employed, she should ask what his job involves, how he travels to it and discover his attitude towards it. Careful observation of the patient's movements, walking, sitting, reaching, etc. will demonstrate any limitation in movement and any groaning or grimacing should be noted. Posture, standing and sitting tolerance should be assessed and his performance noted when he is given a bulky parcel, weighing about 7lbs (3 to 3.5 kg) to lift and carry.

Functional performance must be assessed, noting any difficulty in getting in and out of chair, bed or bath, on and off the toilet and dressing his lower half.

The therapist should ask the patient how his back pain affects his daily life, and she must be prepared to listen. The tale told, and the way it is told, may be very revealing and may enable the therapist to make a psychological assessment of the patient, noting whether he is depressed, angry or frustrated.

The occupational therapist will now be in a position to plan the treatment, which may include:

- instruction in correct posture;
- instruction in lifting techniques;
- advice on back care;
- provision of tools for living;
- possible referral to social worker or clinical psychologist;
- possible referral to Disablement Resettlement Officer.

If the patient's episode of pain is acute in nature, it is wiser to teach proper body mechanics rather than provide tools for living. These tools should be provided only for long-term or recurrent back pain, and then only the minimum tools supplied, as they might reinforce the invalid role. Possible tools include:

- reasonably high chair with good lumbar support;
- firm bed of suitable height;
- work surfaces suited to the patient's height;
- toilet seat raise, toilet frame or handrails;
- long reacher;
- long shoehorn;
- sock or tights aid;
- elastic shoelaces;
- long-handled sponge;
- perching stool to avoid standing for long periods;
- long-handled dustpan and brush;
- long-handled gardening tools.

Advice on back care

The physiotherapist may teach the techniques of lifting and instruct in postural improvement, and the occupational therapist will reinforce and build on this. Lifting is so crucial to the care of the spine that some detail is necessary. To enlarge on the brief mention made in the Pedretti reference:

- Test the object to be lifted. If it is too heavy or awkward, get help.
- Stand with feet apart, the leading foot pointing in the direction of travel.
- Never lift and twist at the same time.

- Bend the knees, using hip and thigh muscles to lift, with the object between the knees.
- Hold load close to the body.
- When rising, 'uncurl' the spine gradually. Do not regain the lumbar lordosis too quickly.

Follow the above sequence in reverse to put an object down.

When lifting with one arm, e.g. a bucket, the above principles should be followed but the free hand must be placed on the bent knee to support the trunk. Lifting above shoulder height increases the lordosis and alters the balance, and lifting an object above head height is even more hazardous. One foot must be placed behind the other and the weight transferred onto the back foot as the object is lifted down. Sturdy steps should be used if possible.

Seating

Sitting imposes additional stress on the spine and low back pain is usually increased by sitting in a low chair with the back bent into a C shape. Firm upholstery is to be preferred. Ideally, a chair should be made to measure and the rules as laid out in Chapter 1 may be followed. There should be enough seat space to enable changing position, as sitting too long in one position will aggravate the pain.

People who sit long hours at a desk need an ergonomically designed chair. The seat height and angle and the backrest angle should be adjustable, and it should be possible to lean forwards over the desk and lean back to talk in a chair which will accommodate both positions. The Droopsnoot does this by virtue of a rocker base. With this chair, as with others with a forward inclining seat, such as the Balans seats, the knees are bent so that the feet are positioned beneath the hips which encourages a good natural position for the spinal curves. The Putnam wedge placed on the chair seat has a similar effect. (Details of suppliers in appendix.)

The desk top should be at elbow height and sloping upwards away from the user, with a holder for copy material, in order to prevent neck strain.

Various portable backrests are available for adapting unsuitable chairs and may be used in cars, at places of entertainment, etc. They usually consist of a moulded framework to support the lumbar curve and should be adjustable. A cheap, simple support may be made with a small towel rolled up or a small cushion lightly filled with polystyrene beads, tucked into the lumbar curve when sitting.

If an existing chair is too low but otherwise supportive, it should be raised from below by one of the methods suggested in Chapter 1.

Sitting with the legs slightly apart puts less stress on the spinal muscles than with the legs together. If suitable clothing is worn, decency need not be sacrificed!

It must be remembered that since back pain has various causes and the individual's build is another variable, the rules regarding seating must remain flexible.

Mattresses

These should be firm but the surface should 'give' a little to accommodate the body contours. If the mattress is too soft, a board must be placed beneath it. The board must be wide enough to allow for rolling over in sleep and should reach from the head to at least below the buttocks.

Patients who are considering buying an 'orthopaedic' mattress should be advised that these are no better than a good quality firm mattress and are more expensive.

Back sufferers will find the use of pillow support helpful, as suggested earlier. In addition, when lying on the side, a pillow in the hollow beneath the waist may help.

Getting out of bed often presents problems. The patient should lie on his side, bend both knees, lower the feet to the floor, at the same time pushing the trunk up with the hand, to prevent lateral flexion or rotation of the spine. The height of the bed should be 20–24 inches (51–61 cm), depending on the individual's height, to enable easy rising.

Bathing

A non-slip mat on the floor of the bath or shower is essential for safety, and a handrail on the wall, at the optimum position for security and support, is desirable. The patient may find he can more easily get in and out of the bath by standing side on to it, bending the nearer knee and lifting the leg sideways over the side of the bath, then repeating the process with the other leg. If the bath is high, a platform may be used with this method.

Patients may be tempted to lie in a warm bath to obtain comfort. The position in which they lie is harmful and causes more pain afterwards. Standing to shower is preferable and the hair may be washed at the same time. If there is no shower, the hair should be washed while kneeling in the bath.

The teeth may be brushed while standing erect. The only time when bending is necessary is when rinsing the mouth and then the hips and knees should do the work.

Dressing

The problems occur when dressing the lower half, and in order to do this it may be more comfortable to stand with the back against a wall and bring the foot up to get clothing on. The foot may be placed on a stool in order to tie the shoelaces. The patient should be reminded not to stretch any elastic laces before tying them in a permanent bow, as there will then be no remaining elasticity to enable easy slipping on and off the shoes. Shoes with a low heel and resilient soles to absorb shock should be worn.

It is important to wear clothing suited to the job in hand. Old or dirty clothing should be worn for handling dirty work, so that items may be held close to the body without fear of spoiling clothing.

Housework

Back pain is a good excuse for avoiding this! Long-handled implements should be used where appropriate and an upright vacuum cleaner may be used, walking to and fro with it, not bending either forwards or laterally if suffering an acute episode. To reach under furniture, the patient should kneel on one knee and if 'getting down to the job', he should kneel on a pad, support the body weight with one hand and work with the other. When cleaning windows or otherwise reaching upwards, a sturdy stool should be used and care taken not to over-reach. If a bucket of water is used, it should have the minimum of water in it.

It is wise to get each member of the household to clean the bath after use. It is easier to clean it before getting out, or a good bubble bath will clean both bath and bather.

Use of fitted sheets and duvets make bedmaking simpler. When changing bed linen, the job should be done in the kneeling position and care taken not to reach across a double bed, but to approach the bed from both sides.

Kitchen

Ideally the work surface height should be correct for the height of the individual, with a continuous level surface to include the cooker top so that items may be slid along rather than carried. A high-level oven is to be preferred, otherwise it is necessary to kneel to use the oven. Regularly used items should be stored within easy reach, and turntables inside cupboards or shelves on the inner side of cupboard doors help in this respect.

If standing is painful, a perching stool may be used for preparation of meals but there may then be tension in the back muscles or the patient may well slump into a poor postural position. If the pain is caused by a trapped nerve, the patient may find relief by resting the affected leg on a footstool while standing.

Laundry

If the bowl is not high enough for handwashing in comfort, it may be put on the drainer or placed on a second bowl upturned in the sink. The clothes should be swirled in the water and not lifted up and down, and only a little should be washed at a time. It is necessary to kneel to load a frontloading washing machine. When emptying the machine a basket should stand ready on a stool to receive the washing, and rotating of the trunk during this procedure is to be avoided. The laundry should be wheeled out on a trolley for hanging out and a prop or pulley system used so that the clothes line is not too high.

When ironing, the board should be adjusted to two inches below elbow height and only essential ironing done, a little at a time. A stool or footstool may be used as described for kitchen activities.

Shopping

This should be done a little at a time if possible and the load evenly divided between two bags. A shopping trolley is difficult to unload and dragging it causes rotation stresses on the spine. If the handle is high enough to be pushed without stooping, a trolley is suitable. When shopping by car, the heavier bags should be placed close at the front of the boot and the lighter items further back. The same rules apply to carrying and loading luggage.

Driving

Driving is a major factor in the aggravation of low back pain, especially if the driving seat is poorly designed or the driver is uncomfortable or tense. If the seat is over-hard, every bump or vibration is transmitted up the vertebral column. The backrest should support the lumbar curve, with extra support if necessary. Alternatively, the driving seat may be replaced with a more supportive model. The pedals should be in a direct line with the legs, allowing the heels to rest comfortably on the floor.

To get into a car, the seat should be moved well back. The driver should sit on the seat, bending the hips and knees but maintaining the lumbar curve, and should then bring the legs into the car, avoiding twisting the spine. It may then be necessary to move the seat position forward to reach the controls. On a long journey, the driver should stop and walk about at intervals.

Sport

Injury is less likely to occur if the individual warms up first. Contact sports may be contra-indicated, and golf, tennis serving and cricket bowling involve rotation of the spine. Jogging is contra-indicated, as it jars the spine. Any walking or sporting activity demands that well-padded, resilient shoes are worn in order to absorb shock.

Gardening

When digging (or clearing snow) a small spade should be used, or a small border fork if the soil is heavy clay. The work should be done from the hips and knees, using the body weight to push the spade into the ground and keeping the back straight. Only a little digging should be done at a time and never if the soil is wet. A Terrex spade with a spring-loaded device to ease the work may be used, or the task delegated. Rakes and hoes should be used while standing erect.

Wheelbarrows must be lightly and evenly loaded and the initial lifting and lowering of the handles done by bending the knees. The two-wheeled barrow causes less stress to the spine.

Mowing machines should be pushed forward using the body weight, and hover machines avoided. Hand weeding and planting out should be performed as for floor-level kitchen activities. 'Easi-kneelers' are not helpful to back sufferers, since one has to bend down an extra few inches to reach the ground. Special weeding tools are available, but no one weeder seems to be suited to the uprooting of every type of weed.

Looking after babies and small children

When carrying children, the principles of lifting should be observed. A cot with the sides lowering right down or a bed with cot sides should be used, and the knees and hips bent for lifting the child in and out. Nappies must be changed on a high surface and the same applies to bathing a baby. The bath may be filled and baled out using a jug to avoid heavy lifting, or a Sunflower Shallowbath or similar adaptation used in the bath, while kneeling to bath the child. A toddler can be encouraged to climb onto a designated stool for help with dressing or to be picked up. If a toddler starts to bounce or wriggle while being held, he must be put down.

Caring for the elderly or handicapped

Carers are at risk if they have to turn, lift or carry disabled relatives. This risk increases as the carer grows older and the elderly relative deteriorates or the handicapped child grows. Caring for an orthopaedic patient in plaster is heavy and the patient is unwieldy, so it follows that the carer needs advice and equipment to protect his back, for his own sake and for that of his dependent. A start can be made by advising on equipment for use in the ward, and this can be continued into the home situation. Carers must be taught correct lifting techniques to maintain their own physical fitness by doing exercises for spinal and abdominal muscles and, if they have a back problem, must wear a lumbar support when lifting. They should also be advised on diet for the dependent, to prevent them becoming overweight.

It is important that bed, chair, commode or toilet heights are the same to enable sliding transfers without having to lift. A turntable also helps with transfers and a monkey pole over the bedhead enables the dependent person to help himself. A hoist may be provided after careful assessment and instruction in use. Simpler lifting aids are available including the patient handling sling, which in effect lengthens the carer's arms so that he can keep his back straighter when reaching forward to lift.

Sexual problems

Sexual problems are usually due to pain but complaining of back pain may be an excuse to avoid sexual activity. Anxiety or depression may cause inability to achieve an erection, producing further anxiety. This may require counselling and possible medication.

The pain problem may be overcome by:

- a simple analgesic half an hour before intercourse;
- use of a firm mattress, with a pillow under the lumbar spine;
- possible reversal of traditional male and female positions;
- the woman on all fours, with her partner approaching from behind;
- the man sitting on a chair with his partner sitting astride him;
- both partners lying on their sides.

If sexual intercourse is too painful and frustrating after these suggestions have been tried, it may be preferable for the couple to concentrate on other aspects of loving intimacy.

A booklet incorporating the foregoing, from 'Advice on Back Care' onwards, may be drawn up and given to patients to remind them to take continuing responsibility for their own back care.

REFERENCES AND FURTHER READING

See lists following Chapter 6.

6

Spinal surgery

Spinal surgery is performed on only four patients in every 10,000 recorded attacks of low back pain (Jayson, 1987). Conservative treatment is always tried first.

Criteria for spinal surgery include:

- radiological evidence of loss of disc space;
- persistent sciatica;
- persistent neurological signs, with muscular weakness and loss of tendon reflexes;
- progressive spinal abnormality and deformity;
- disease such as TB or tumour.

It is useful for the occupational therapist to know in broad outline what is involved in the most frequently performed spinal operations.

DISCECTOMY

The more usual discectomy procedure is the removal of the whole disc to prevent recurrence, although if most of the disc is in place, the protruding piece only may be removed along with any loose fragments of cartilage. If the vertebra is likely to displace, the surgeon will perform a spinal fusion between the vertebrae adjacent to the discectomy. The patient may then wear a lumbar corset for a few weeks post-operatively. He may return to work within four to six weeks, or three months if his work is heavy.

Decompression

If spinal canal stenosis is caused by a disc protrusion, discectomy is performed. This may be accompanied by decompression to widen the spinal canal and prevent pressure on a nerve root. Small pieces of bone are removed to widen the spinal canal. There are two types of decompression:

1. laminectomy, with partial or complete removal of the lamina of the vertebra;
2. facetectomy, where bone is removed from the inner edge of the facet joint.

The patient begins to mobilize two to three days after surgery, and is discharged after seven to ten days. He must avoid lifting and strenuous exercise for three months.

SPINAL FUSION

This operation is carried out if there is excessive mobility in the lumbar spine or if there is facet joint damage. The latter may be caused by spinal degeneration, failed back surgery or as a later result of disc trauma. Spinal fusion is performed to relieve spondylolisthesis, where the misaligned vertebrae are damaging nerves, causing pain, numbness and tingling in the legs. It is also the procedure used to treat the TB spine.

There are differing techniques for the operation, as surgeons develop their own methods (Figure 6.1). One is the interbody fusion where the disc space is

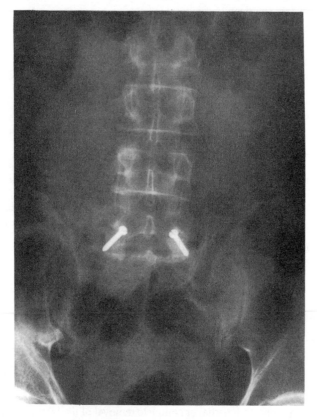

Figure 6.1 Alzar spinal fusion

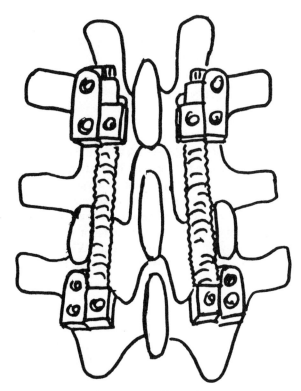

Figure 6.2 Posterior segment fixator *in situ*

filled with bone chippings, usually from the ilium. Another is the posterolateral fusion, in which slivers of bone from the ilium are placed over the facet joints between the transverse process, on one or both sides of the vertebrae. A third technique is the spinal fusion done in two stages: the first a posterior fusion, then if this is considered to be insufficiently stable, an anterior fusion is performed a few weeks later.

Post-operatively the patient is on bedrest for two weeks or more, then may wear a plaster cast or corset for six to eight weeks. It takes about six to 12 months for the patient to feel the full benefit from the operation. Because the fusion has reduced movement in one area, the adjacent joints will be more stressed. Adhesions may result from post-operative inflammation. This may result in chronic back pain.

The posterior segment fixator (PSF) for the spine aims to reduce intervertebral deformity by means of screws anchored in the vertebrae through the pedicles (Figure 6.2). This stabilizes the vertebral segments and allows early mobilization without the need for external back supports. The device may be used to correct spinal instability, scoliosis, infections, tumours, spondylolisthesis and may act as a stabilizer while healing takes place following spinal fusion. It may be left in situ or removed at a later date.

INSERTION OF A HARRINGTON ROD

This operation is one which is performed for severe scoliosis, usually in an adolescent. For the whole length of the scoliosis, the spinous processes are removed and the outer layers of bone chipped back to form flaps. A telescopic Harrington rod is inserted to open up the curve for distraction on the concave side, and another rod may be used for compression on the convex side. Chips of bone, usually from the ilium, are laid along the curved section and the bone flaps turned down over them. The patient is discharged after two to three weeks, and is off work for another month. He must avoid sports for six to 12 months. The rods are removed later, when the fusion is solid. While this surgery improves the patient's appearance, it does result in a very stiff back.

HALO TRACTION

This is sometimes used in the treatment of scoliosis or as a form of splinting following spinal fusion. It consists of a metal 'halo' round the skull penetrating the outer part of the skull by means of four screws, with four distraction bars connecting the halo to a pelvic hoop which is held by two pins inserted through the ilium and sacrum. Distraction proceeds at the rate of 1 mm per day. Spring balances on the distraction bars record the pressures very carefully. The patient is carefully monitored for signs of double vision, neck pain, pain in limbs or around the screw holes in the skull, sensory abnormalities and muscle weakness.

The patient is encouraged in personal independence. The most obvious precaution is to remind the patient to pay attention to his unaccustomed height when going through doors, otherwise a very unpleasant and possibly damaging jolt will occur.

The use of a monkey pole is contra-indicated in this case.

POST-OPERATIVE PRECAUTIONS AFTER SPINAL SURGERY

The immediate precautions are rest, and probably wearing a back support when mobile. The longer term precautions are covered by 'Care of the Spine' in Chapter 5. The patient who has had any kind of spinal surgery should be encouraged to think positively, to accept that the cause of his back pain has been dealt with, and to work towards a normal lifestyle, while taking sensible precautions.

The physiotherapist teaches the patient how to get in and out of bed, in the method described in the previous chapter. When on bedrest the patient may usually lie in the position he finds most comfortable, provided the spine is not rotated. A pillow between the knees when side-lying and/or a pillow under the waist curve will help to prevent undesirable positions. When rolling over, the patient should turn the whole body, head and legs in one smooth movement. If the facet joints are involved, lying prone is uncomfortable and lying on the back increases the lordosis, causing pain. Lying on the side with hips and knees bent approximately at right angles is more comfortable.

As the patient starts to mobilize, the physiotherapist encourages him to 'walk tall' and to concentrate on his posture. Short walks are gradually lengthened as strength returns, and after exercise the patient lies on the bed to rest. No walking aids are used. Standing is avoided in the early days.

Sitting is delayed until seven days post-operatively, and for three to four weeks in the case of spinal fusion. At first the patient sits just to eat meals, gradually progressing to longer periods in a chair. Sitting up in bed with the legs outstretched is not allowed. Crossing the legs is contra-indicated, as this causes a tilted pelvis, spinal imbalance, compression of the discs and possible pressure on a nerve root on the side to which the leg is crossed.

Surgical corsets and spinal supports

Since a significant proportion of patients are fitted with spinal supports immediately following surgery, and since the wearing of these supports has some bearing on the daily living activities of the patient, it is useful for the occupational therapist to know the theory behind this provision and the types of support which may be used.

The purpose of the corseting is to restrict movements of the lumbar spine to allow healing to proceed, and to encourage use of the hips and knees for bending activity. 'Off-the-peg' corsets have no place in this context, as they never fit properly.

The types of back support include:

1. Corsets made to measure. These include corsets with a pocket enclosing a mouldable panel, which is moulded to the patient's back in the same way as for splinting a hand, with the patient lying prone.
2. Neofract moulded jackets with a zipped fastening, so they are removable for bathing or lying down. They have the advantage of being rigid and really supportive without the weight and bulk of plaster of Paris.
3. Plaster of Paris cast. This is sometimes applied after spinal fusion. It restricts movement for 24 hours a day and is worn for approximately six to eight weeks. It is heavy and claustrophobic.

When a patient is wearing any of these supports, it is apparent that when he sits down, the corset/support is pushed up. This is especially obvious with the plaster cast, and some of these are moulded in a vest-like shape, which may push up almost to the patient's ears. Not surprisingly, the patient is depressed by this cumbersome and ugly contraption and needs much encouragement and some suggestions as to how to minimize the problems it causes. Not least of these problems is the frequently encountered one of toilet hygiene, because the patient cannot twist to reach the anal area. It is important that an efficient tool is provided so he can maintain his independence in this most intimate task. A sponge on an angled handle approximately nine inches long, with a slit in the sponge on the outer rim to slot in the ends of the toilet paper, is helpful. The shorter of the long-handled sponges commercially available is suitable.

During the wearing of a spinal support, the patient is doing static exercises to strengthen his spinal extensors and abdominal muscles. The support is a means to an end and should be worn for a limited period, as prescribed by the surgeon. If it is worn for too long, the patient's musculature becomes dependent on it and these soft tissues weaken and become ineffective, leading to collapse of the spine. Once the prescribed period for wearing the support has expired, the corset should be dispensed with so that the muscles and ligaments may take over their normal function. A corset may be retained to wear intermittently, when doing heavier work, undertaking prolonged activity, during a long car journey, or to use briefly during an acute episode.

OCCUPATIONAL THERAPY

The aims and objectives of both physiotherapy and occupational therapy are similar to those listed under the Back School concept in Chapter 5.

Use of correct seating with adequate spinal support is important. To rise from his chair, the patient should move forward in the seat and push upwards and forwards with the hands from the chair arms, maintaining the lumbar curve. If rising from a chair without arms, 'walking' the hands up the front of the thighs may facilitate standing. The patient should stand up straight before starting to walk.

Once the patient is able to use the ward toilet, the occupational therapist should ascertain whether he needs any toilet aids on discharge. Such provision will depend on what type of surgery has been performed, the patient's height, age, and whether he is wearing any spinal support. He should try out toilet aids so that he is familiar with their use. Any necessary equipment should be requisitioned from the community agency in time for it to be fitted in readiness for the patient's discharge.

Bending down is avoided for at least four weeks in the case of spinal fusion, much longer if bone grafting has been employed, possibly less in the case of decompression. The surgeon will advise the patient on this, depending on the surgical technique adopted. Meanwhile the patient is encouraged to get used to bending from the hips and knees instead. A long reacher is needed from the outset for spinal fusion patients, and may be in use for many weeks. Most patients will be independent in dressing by their discharge date, using a long reacher for putting on pants and trousers, and if sciatic pain was present before surgery, the leg in which this pain was experienced should be put into the pants first. Putting socks or tights on while lying on the bed may preclude the use of aids.

If the patient is wearing a plaster cast he will be limited in what clothing he can wear, as his girth will be much increased by the bulk of the plaster. Track suits are useful as they are loose fitting and are relatively inexpensive. Some patients may need referral to the social worker for help in purchasing larger sizes in clothing.

Tools for living

Similar items to those listed for back pain will be needed. The need for equipment is greater than for back pain which has been conservatively treated, but the patient is given to understand that the equipment will be needed for a limited period, until healing has taken place.

If a chair is obtained for a patient on short term loan, he should be made aware that while he is borrowing this chair he should be taking steps to obtain a suitable chair for himself for permanent use. The necessary information for doing this is best provided in an information sheet after verbal and/or practical instruction.

A flow chart is useful to monitor achievement of objectives (Figure 6.3).

So far we have considered only pain in the lumbosacral area. The occupational therapist's services are also needed after surgery to the cervical spine and the coccyx.

CERVICAL SPINE

Neck postural pain due to work at a desk with the head bent for long periods, possibly with the shoulders hunched, leads to chronic muscular tension. Advice on suitable office furniture may be given, as discussed in Chapter 5.

Facet joint problems in the cervical spine cause aching and sharp twinges of pain, with pins and needles or numbness in the hands and possibly loss of balance, headache, tinnitus and referred pain in the side of the face, ear or neck.

Vertebro-basilar insufficiency is due to vertebral artery compression, probably caused by osteophytes giving rise to spinal canal stenosis. Turning the head or stretching the neck then causes giddiness or blackouts.

Brachialgia is caused by protrusion of a cervical disc pressing on a nerve

OCCUPATIONAL THERAPY DEPARTMENT SP. SURG.

NAME:

NUMBER:

DATE:

Pre-Op	Op.	Day 1	Day 2	Day 3	Day 4	Day 5	Day 6	Day 7	Day 8	Day 9	Day 10	Day 11	Day 12	Day 13 etc
Introduce self, check home situation, help, accom, etc			As pre-op if not already done. Loan H/Hand	→										
						When pt. up to W.C. assess needs →								
							Monitor progress			∧				
								Discuss ADL solutions and precautions incl. work →		Dressing practice lower half Tools needed? →				∧
								Preliminary referral to supplier of equipment →		Detailed referral plus expected discharge date →			∧	Check equipment delivered and fitted
														Teach technique for in\out of bath

Figure 6.3 Flow chart for monitoring achievement of objectives following spinal surgery

root, producing severe pain down the arm to the hand, possibly with numbness or pins and needles. There may also be upper limb weakness.

Patients with rheumatoid arthritis with instability of the atlanto-axial joint may present with symptoms of spinal cord compression, causing neurological signs in the lower limbs, e.g. spasticity, sensory loss or incontinence.

Patients with any of the conditions listed above, with the exception of postural pain, may require a cervical collar to provide support, reduce pressure and prevent undesirable movement. This will relieve pain and allow inflammation to subside. Standard collars are adequate in mild cases but a moulded collar in thermoplastic splinting material or block leather may be indicated, which may be fitted by the orthotist, physiotherapist or occupational therapist. The aim is to achieve a closely fitting, highly supportive splint to prevent movement of the cervical spine. While there is some controversy over this, it should reach from the occipital condyles down to the seventh cervical vertebra or lower at the back, and support the chin and reach to the manubrium sterni at the front. Depending on the surgeon's directions, the patient will wear the collar for 24 hours a day or during the day only, for a variable length of time. It should be discarded gradually, but retained for use on car journeys. In cases of instability of the atlanto-axial joint, the collar is worn until the instability is resolved and not discarded until the surgeon has confirmed that it is safe to do so.

The patient may be more comfortable when lying down if the pillow is twisted in the middle to form a 'butterfly' to stabilize the neck. Various pillows, shaped to accommodate the cervical curve, are available. Alternatively, a small towel may be rolled up and wrapped around the neck at night.

Fusion of the cervical spine may be unavoidable. The operation carries some risk of paraplegia or even death. A neurosurgeon is therefore often called in to perform the surgery. Post-operatively the patient is discharged after about four to ten days wearing a rigid collar. He may be able to return to work in a month at the surgeon's discretion, or after two months if his work involves lifting or driving.

COCCYDINIA

This is due to a fall onto the coccyx. It is very painful and may persist for a long time. An injection of lignocaine or marcaine may relieve the pain, but occasionally surgery is necessary.

Coccygectomy involves the removal of the last two or three segments of the coccyx. In the case of non-union of a fractured coccyx the fragment is removed. Post-operatively the patient is up in a few days and may return to work in two to three weeks.

The main problem before and immediately after surgery is sitting comfortably. An anti-pressure type cushion may be needed to disperse the load, or a cushion provided with a channel running centrally from front to back, so that there is a space beneath the coccyx. If the patient finds bending is also painful, he may need a reaching tool for a few weeks.

In over 30% of cases, surgery fails to relieve low back pain and many patients seek further surgery (Cailliet, 1988). If the patient's pain continues for over six months, chronic back pain is considered to have developed, although Cailliet writes that some authorities consider that six weeks of persistent pain constitutes chronic pain. The aim in the treatment of low back pain is to prevent development of chronic pain syndrome, because of its high emotional cost to the patient and his family and the high financial cost to the employer and the cost of health care. The occupational therapist has much to offer in the prevention and treatment of this syndrome, and this is discussed in Chapter 11.

REFERENCES FOR CHAPTERS 5 AND 6

Cailliet R. (1988) *Low Back Pain Syndrome*, F.A. Davis, Philadelphia.

Jayson, M.V. (1987) *Back Pain: The facts*, 2nd edn, Oxford Medical Publications, Oxford.

Pedretti, L.W. (1981) *Occupational Therapy Practice Skills for Physical Dysfunction*, Mosby, St Louis.

Tanner, J. (1987) *Beating Back Pain*, Dorling Kindersley, London.

FURTHER READING

Mounayer, B. and Wyn-Williams, S. (1989) *The Back Shop Book*, Macdonald, London.

Willer, A.P. and Rowland, D. (1985) *Back to Backs*. Published by the authors, available from Wimbledon Physiotherapy Clinic, 28a Wilton Grove, London SW19 3QX.

7

Shoulder surgery

By comparison with hip and knee surgery, relatively few operations have been performed on the shoulder. Those which have have been mainly for repair of fractures of the proximal humerus, and for rheumatoid and osteo-arthritis of the shoulder joint.

THE ROTATOR CUFF

At the glenohumeral joint, movement takes place between the humerus and scapula, and between the scapula and chest wall, when the arm is abducted. The stability of the joint depends largely on the muscles and tendons surrounding it, the tendons being inserted into the tuberosities of the humeral head. The tendons involved are subscapularis anteriorly, and supraspinatus, infraspinatus and teres minor posteriorly, and these blend with and reinforce the joint capsule. Collectively they are referred to as the rotator cuff.

In the event of a fall, the rotator cuff is vulnerable and there may be extensive damage, depending on the direction of the fall. The most likely tendon to be torn is that of the supraspinatus resulting in the inability to initiate abduction, although once the arm is passively abducted, the deltoid takes over in raising the arm. Following a tear in the rotator cuff, rest is usually recommended for a short period, then mobilization commenced quickly to prevent stiffness developing. Repair surgery is possible but tricky. Lesions of the rotator cuff are significant in the prognosis following shoulder replacement.

If conservative treatment for glenohumeral arthritis fails, any of the following operations may be considered:

1. total shoulder replacement;
2. hemi-arthroplasty;
3. arthrodesis.

TOTAL SHOULDER ARTHROPLASTY

This operation involves the replacement of the humeral head and the resurfacing of the glenoid cavity. There are constrained, unconstrained and semi-constrained types of prostheses.

The constrained prosthesis consists of a linked ball and socket joint which produces a rotating unit but does not allow for the small amount of shift that occurs during rotation, when the humeral head moves upwards in the glenoid cavity. On abduction the head of the humerus descends in the glenoid cavity. The glenohumeral joint is therefore a minimally constrained joint with a wide range of mobility, depending largely for its stability on the muscles of the shoulder girdle. The constrained prosthesis therefore limits the restoration of mobility, and there is a tendency for the glenoid component to loosen. Initially

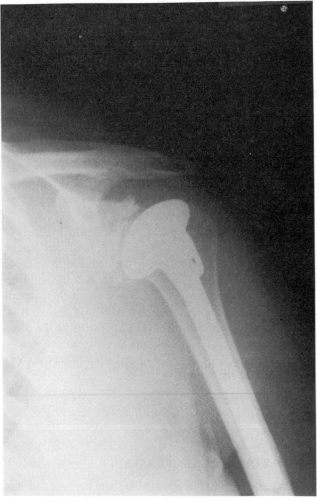

Figure 7.1 Neer II total shoulder replacement

pain relief is good but once the prosthesis loosens, pain recurs. The Stanmore prosthesis is an example of a more constrained arthroplasty. If the rotator cuff is damaged, a constrained prosthesis must be used.

An unconstrained arthroplasty depends for its stability on an intact rotator cuff. The prosthesis consists of a metal humeral component and a glenoid component with a keel for fixation. The glenoid component is of high-density polyethylene, or metal-backed high-density polyethylene, cemented in place. The Neer II prosthesis is an example and more nearly resembles the natural shoulder joint (Figure 7.1). The unconstrained type may become semi-constrained by using a glenoid component with a lip posteriorly, to resist subluxation when the arm is abducted.

A survey of 70 total shoulder replacements conducted in Ontario, Canada, demonstrated that with both rheumatoid and osteo-arthritis, pain relief was satisfactory in approximately 90% of patients. Both groups achieved increased range of movement but the improvement was greater with the osteo-arthritis group (Hawkins *et al.*, 1989). If the rotator cuff is intact, the patient can expect to gain forward flexion and elevation beyond 90°, and considerably more if he had osteo-arthritis. On average, range of movement post-operatively is 50–65% of normal with rheumatoid disease and 75–80% of normal with osteo-arthritis.

Later, loosening of the glenoid component or dislocation may occur with a constrained prosthesis. With unconstrained prostheses, later complications may include glenoid component loosening or wearing, dislocation, humeral component loosening or rotator cuff tear. A severely disabled patient with rheumatoid arthritis who has to use crutches will increase the stresses on the shoulder and exacerbate the problem of loosening (Souter, 1987).

Removal of the humeral component for revision is difficult, but is rarely necessary. Revision of the glenoid component is more likely, and if the bone stock is poor, may necessitate bone grafting. The prosthesis can be expected to last for many years, especially with patients with rheumatoid disease who have more restricted mobility.

Rehabilitation for total shoulder replacement

Aims and objectives are broadly as those following hip replacement.

The muscles of the shoulder girdle are likely to have atrophied due to disuse prior to surgery, so rehabilitation is aimed at building up these muscles and mobilizing the shoulder joint. Depending on the surgeon's preference, passive exercises by the physiotherapist are started on the second to fifth post-operative day, aiming at forward elevation and external rotation, with internal rotation a little later. Most patients are discharged one or two weeks after surgery but attend for physiotherapy for another two months. They progress through passive and assisted to active movement, and are also expected to perform exercises at home. Most authorities recommend pendulum exercises and shoulder shrugging. Around four to six weeks post-operatively, patients are given resisted exercise. The supporting sling may be discarded at any time from one week after surgery, once the patient is comfortable.

Daily living activities

Because the patient had restricted movement and pain prior to admission, he may already have appropriate tools for living. The type of tools he now needs include:

- long angled-handle sponge and comb;
- Manoy or other rocker knife;
- Dycem matting;
- dressing stick;
- front-fastening clothing of loose fit.

Because he can use his hand, the patient may be able to perform most two-handed tasks provided shoulder elevation is not needed. Dressing the affected arm first and undressing it last may need to be reinforced. Kitchen activity incorporating the principles of joint protection must be undertaken (see Chapter 1).

The patient should be encouraged to discard tools for living gradually as he becomes able. In the long term, a patient who has had shoulder arthroplasty should avoid heavy lifting, tugging and jerky movements, and any extreme movements which force the joint. Sports, such as golf, should also be avoided.

CUP ARTHROPLASTY

This operation may be used for rheumatoid patients. A hemispherical stainless steel cup is cemented onto the prepared humeral head. Its advantage is that it does not damage the medullary cavity of the humerus, and may be converted to a total arthroplasty or to arthrodesis in the event of failure.

HEMI-ARTHROPLASTY

This is replacement of the humeral head and may be used for patients with rheumatoid or osteo-arthritis of the shoulder. However, the articulation between the metal humeral head and the bone of the glenoid eventually wears away the cartilage and then causes bony erosion, so the long term effects are disappointing. The principles of bipolar arthroplasty may overcome this problem (Figure 7.2). A clinical comparison between the results of hemi-arthroplasty and total arthroplasty (Bell and Gschwend, 1986) reported that, in a trial group, 59% of hemi-arthroplasties were satisfactory but the remaining 41% still had a painful

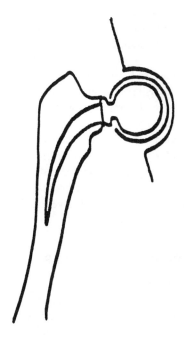

Figure 7.2 Principle of bipolar arthroplasty

shoulder, while the range of movement was significantly better in the group who had had total arthroplasty.

Physiotherapy aims to achieve maximum possible mobility. Passive and then assisted exercises are carefully increased as tolerated. The patient is taught exercises to perform at home, or may attend as an outpatient for up to eight weeks post-operatively. Pendulum exercises are typical during this period. If the tuberosities on the humeral head are intact, exercises for muscle strength may be commenced about two weeks after surgery.

The movements required to perform daily living tasks are forward elevation and internal and external rotation, particularly necessary for dressing and grooming. For the first few weeks patients may need some assistance in these tasks. As function improves, they must be encouraged to use the joint to its maximum potential.

SHOULDER ARTHRODESIS

This operation is more rarely encountered as methods of shoulder arthroplasty improve. It is more useful for osteo-arthritic shoulders, as it affords pain relief and reasonable function. It is a less satisfactory procedure for rheumatoid shoulders, as multiple joints are involved. The shoulder is fixed in approximately 30–45° of abduction, 20° of flexion and 15° of external rotation, which is a good functional position. The shoulder is immobilized in a shoulder spica plaster for three months until union is sound, after which the physiotherapist starts to re-educate the scapular muscles for compensatory movement.

While the patient is in plaster, he will need a number of tools for living. The bulky plaster necessitates larger size clothing, which should be of a stretchy fabric, with few fastenings. The dressing method of the affected arm into the clothing first and out last must be adopted. Because the hand is in an elevated position, the only way the two hands can be used together will be in an unnatural position. Tools such as Dycem matting, rocker knife, plate bunker and wire saucepan basket are necessary. The patient should practise opening jars by holding them steady between the knees, and straining vegetables either into a colander in the sink or through a wire saucepan basket.

RECURRENT DISLOCATION OF THE SHOULDER

This is often the result of a sports injury to a young man, and is apt to dislocate on abduction and external rotation. The usual operation is the Putti-Platt procedure, in which the range of external rotation is limited by taking a tuck in the anterior joint capsule and another tuck in the subscapularis tendon. After surgery, the patient has his arm bound to his side for six weeks, before gentle mobilization is commenced. The condition also occurs in female patients with congenital joint laxity, but instead of surgery patients are advised to restrict their physical activity.

FRACTURES OF THE PROXIMAL HUMERUS

While these fractures come under the category of trauma rather than cold orthopaedics, they do on occasion appear on the orthopaedic ward. These fractures are quite common in older people and are caused by a fall on the outstretched arm. C.S.Neer, the surgeon who pioneered the Neer shoulder replacement, classified humeral fractures into seven groups:

1. Undisplaced fractures, which heal after immobilization in a collar and cuff sling.
2. Fracture through the anatomical neck (rare).
3. Fracture through the surgical neck, with rotator cuff unimpaired.
4. Fracture of the greater tuberosity, with rotator cuff ruptured.
5. Fracture of the lesser tuberosity, possibly also including displacement of the surgical neck, and possibly involving the greater tuberosity.
6. Fracture dislocation, when the head of the humerus may be separated from

its blood supply. There may also be involvement of the brachial plexus and axillary blood vessels.

7. Fractures involving the articular surfaces.

Treatment of these fractures varies according to the fracture site. In most cases, some surgery is required. Where blood supply to the humeral head is lost, a hemi-arthroplasty is performed. This applies to group two, the complex cases in group five, some of group six, and group seven where over 50% of damage is done to the joint surfaces. Treatment by internal fixation applies to groups three, four, five and six if the blood supply to the humeral head is unimpaired, and in group seven when there is 20–50% damage to the joint surfaces.

REMEDIAL OCCUPATIONAL THERAPY FOLLOWING SHOULDER SURGERY

The aims of occupational therapy are:

* to ensure the patient's independence in ADL;
* to encourage perseverance in the rehabilitation programme;
* to improve muscle power and range of movement.

Following a programme of remedial therapy, the patient is expected:

* to be independent in all necessary areas of ADL;
* to understand the precautions necessary for protection of the prosthesis;
* to have full functional use of the affected joint.

The normal range of movement for the shoulder joint is forward flexion 180°, extension 60°, horizontal abduction up to 120° when external rotation enables abduction to continue up to 180°, adduction with some flexion to 45°, external rotation to 80–90° and internal rotation to 70–80°. The last two may be measured functionally by asking the patient to reach the back of his head (external rotation) and putting his forearm along the back of his waist (internal rotation). Alternatively, the elbow may be held close to the trunk, flexed to 90°, and the degree of forearm movements measured outwards (external rotation) and across the trunk (internal rotation).

Should the patient be referred for remedial treatment, close cooperation with physiotherapy is essential. Initially activities should be light and working in the inner range of movement, progressing towards the outer range (i.e. the more extreme limits of movement).

Sample treatment programme

The patient should face the work and be far enough away from it so that he does not substitute elbow and forearm movement for the shoulder exercise. The programme may be commenced 12 days post-operatively if the tuberosities, rotator cuff and glenoid were intact, or six weeks post-operatively if any were damaged prior to surgery.

1. Initially support the forearm in a suspension sling and roll putty to and fro on a level surface. After two days, discard sling to work.
2. Work on an inclined surface, at 20°, rolling putty, polishing wood, playing solitaire, etc.
3. As (2), gradually increasing angle of work surface.
4. Substitute sanding for polishing.
5. Stack lightweight blocks and build towers of stacking discs.
6. Walk the fingers up a small ladder with numbered rungs. Measure progress by the number of the rung reached.
7. As (5), gradually increasing the weight of the blocks and discs.
8. Use of guillotine and printing press, standing to use guillotine.
9. Use of guillotine, cutting thicker card, progressing to sitting to use guillotine.

The above activity aims for forward flexion. At the same time, rotation of the shoulder is obtained by:

1. Manoeuvring a wire maze to get a bead from one side to the other.
2. Building towers of discs, picking up the discs with the elbow extended and forearm pronated, turning them over, and putting them down with the forearm supinated.
3. Grasping a baton with both hands close together and elbows extended, and twisting it clockwise and anti-clockwise. Grade by using heavier batons.

During the first 2–6 weeks, depending on the pre-operative state of the joint, the patient must be warned not to lean on the operated arm. The treatment programme should be carried out in 5–10 minute sessions, preferably for four sessions daily. The patient is discharged three weeks after surgery, but treatment may be continued for up to eight weeks, or more if the rotator cuff was previously damaged.

Care must be taken not to stress the joint unduly. Once adequate range of movement and power for the functions required for the patient's lifestyle have been achieved, it is advisable to stop pushing for too much improvement, as this could shorten the life of the prosthesis.

LIMB LENGTHENING

The methods described for leg lengthening in Chapter 4 are also employed in the treatment of arm length discrepancy. This deformity hinders a child from participation in school sports, among other activities. During the wearing of the fixation device on the humerus, dressing and feeding present problems. Loose clothing with baggy or batwing sleeves with elasticated cuffs are warm and comfortable. Sleeveless tops can be adapted by opening the side seam on the same side as the arm lengthening and attaching velcro dabs. Dungarees and pinafore skirts provide extra winter warmth. Capes are a good substitute for coats. The arm with the Ilizarov frame on will have to be put into garments first when dressing, and last out when undressing. The Disabled Living Foundation Clothing and Footwear Advisory Service is a useful source of information and provide a list of workshops which will alter clothes and may make some garments to order.

Feeding difficulties may be present regardless of whether the dominant or non-dominant arm is being treated, and a Manoy or Nelson knife or a Splayd may be useful. The arm wearing the frame may be used to stabilize a plate, but a plate guard or a Dycem mat may facilitate eating.

REFERENCES

Bell, S.N. and Gschwend, N. (1986) Clinical experience with total arthroplasty and hemi-arthroplasty of the shoulder using the Neer prosthesis, *International Orthopaedics*, **10**, 217–22.

Hawkins, R.J., Bell, R.H. and Jallay, B. (1989) Total shoulder arthroplasty, *Clinical Orthopaedics and Related Research*, **242**, 188–94.

FURTHER READING

Browne, P.S.H. (1985) *Basic Facts in Orthopaedics*, 2nd edn, Blackwell Scientific Publications, Oxford.

Cofield, R.H. and Edgerton, B.C. (1990) *Total Shoulder Arthroplasty: Complications and revision surgery*, Instructional Course Lectures, American Academy of Orthopaedic Surgeons, Chicago.

Hughes, S. (1989) *A New Short Textbook of Orthopaedics and Traumatology*, Edward Arnold, London.

Jonsson, E. *et al.* (1986) Cup arthroplasty of the rheumatoid shoulder, *Acta Orthop Scand*, **57**, 542–6.

Mills, D. and Fraser, C. (1989) *Therapeutic Activities for the Upper Limb*, Winslow Press, Bicester.

Naylor, A. (1955) *Fractures and Orthopaedic Surgery for Nurses and Physiotherapists*, E. and S. Livingstone Ltd, Edinburgh.

Post, M. (1988) *The Shoulder: Surgical and nonsurgical management*, 2nd edn, Lea and Febiger, Philadelphia.

Souter, W.A. (1987) Surgical management of rheumatoid arthritis, in S.P.F. Hughes, M.K. Benson and C. Colton (eds.) *Orthopaedics: The principles and practice of musculoskeletal surgery*, Churchill Livingstone, Edinburgh.

Thornhill, T.S. and Barrett, W.P. (1988) Total shoulder arthroplasty, in C.R. Rowe (ed.) *The Shoulder*, Churchill Livingstone, Edinburgh.

Trombly, C. (1983) *Occupational Therapy for Physical Dysfunction*, Williams and Wilkins, Baltimore.

Watson, M. (1988) Letter on shoulder replacement in *British Medical Journal*, **296,** 1346–7.

8

Elbow surgery

In the elbow joint the main articulation is between the humerus and ulna, at which flexion and extension occur. The radius articulates with the humerus only in flexion. Within the single joint capsule is a separate pivot joint, the proximal radio-ulnar joint. This functions with the distal radio-ulnar joint at the wrist to rotate the forearm. When the elbow is fully extended with the palm facing anteriorly, the forearm is slightly abducted on the humerus, giving rise to the carrying angle.

The complexity and unique construction of the elbow has meant that research into elbow arthroplasty has lagged behind that for the joints of the lower limb. Perhaps for this reason some surgeons still advocate synovectomy for treatment of the rheumatoid elbow. While this affords only minor improvement in range of movement, it gives dramatic pain relief and induces a remission which can last from three to five years (Souter, 1987).

TOTAL ELBOW REPLACEMENT

Types of elbow replacement include the older semi-constrained prosthesis with metal components and a high density polyethylene hinge, and the improved unconstrained prosthesis with one metal and one polyethylene component, designed to resurface the joint. The Souter-Strathclyde and the Wadsworth total elbow arthroplasties are the most frequently used in the United Kingdom. The Souter-Strathclyde (Figure 8.1) is closely modelled on the normal anatomy of the trochlear joint on the anterior aspect of the ulna, with a stirrup-shaped humeral component with a wide area of fixation. The ulna component is a dovetailed keel in the olecranon process, and a short stem into the medullary cavity of the ulna (Souter, 1987). The Wadsworth prosthesis is indicated where there is excessive bone loss or very porotic bone, as it has a longer stem.

These unconstrained prostheses imply the provision of some rotation and laxity of the joint. Improvements continue to be made, with the aim of biological fixation rather than cement, in the hope of reducing the risk of loosening.

Indications for total elbow replacement are pain, instability and loss of function. Suitable candidates are patients with rheumatoid destruction of the elbow and those suffering from post-traumatic osteo-arthritis of the elbow. In

99

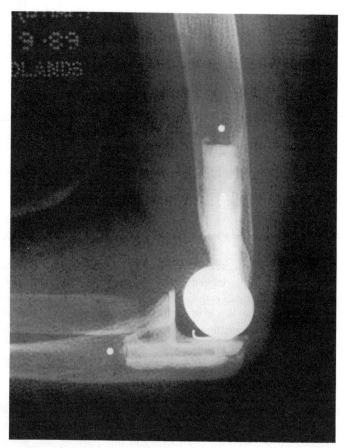

Figure 8.1 Souter-Strathclyde total elbow replacement

the case of the patient with rheumatoid arthritis, careful timing of surgery is important. Any surgery for reconstruction of the joints of the lower limb should be performed first, to prevent stress on the elbow by the use of crutches. Total elbow arthroplasty is contra-indicated in patients with infected joints.

Post-operatively the physio- and occupational therapist have considerable input. Initially the elbow joint is rested for five days. This period may vary according to the surgeon's opinion. Then gentle flexion, extension, pronation and supination exercises are commenced. Between exercise sessions the elbow is rested and supported in an elbow splint with the joint flexed at 90°. Exercise is gradually built up over a six week period, when the splint is discarded and light function is commenced.

OCCUPATIONAL THERAPY FOLLOWING TOTAL ELBOW REPLACEMENT

The aims and objectives of treatment are similar to those for hip replacement.

In the immediate post-operative period, if the patient lives alone he will need items such as a Manoy knife or Splayd fork, dressing stick, long-handled comb and front-fastening clothing. He will also need kitchen practice to familiarize him with using the unoperated arm to handle kettles, saucepans and cooking pots.

Tools for living

The occupational therapist must assess the patient's ability to rise from his chair, bed and toilet, without having to lever himself up with his arms. If she finds he has to use his arms for any of these activities, appropriate equipment should be provided, which may include:

- high seat chair, or raising blocks or other device to raise existing chair;
- spring-lift chair, if rising problems are severe;
- raised toilet seat;
- bedraising blocks;
- bath aids, to prevent levering up from the base of the bath;
- a second stair-rail, so that the patient can use the unoperated arm to hold the stair-rail for climbing and descending stairs;
- if the patient has to depend on the stair-rail, referral for a stairlift.

Force is exerted on the elbow joint when lifting or carrying a heavy object and when leaning on the hand. Torsional stress on the long lever of the forearm occurs when a person works with the shoulder abducted. These actions should therefore be avoided following elbow replacement. Any weight carried should not exceed 1 kg (2.2 lbs) for two to three months post-operatively, then gradually increasing the weight permitted up to a maximum of 5 kg. Therefore, the patient must be educated in ways of avoiding heavy lifting and carrying, e.g. walking to and fro to carry several light loads. Provision of an Etwall trolley enables the patient to wheel heavier objects around, if there are no thresholds or steps in the way. A shopping trolley saves carrying but entails dragging a heavy weight and this, coupled with hauling it up kerbs, produces unacceptable stress on the elbow. A push-type trolley is satisfactory. Pressure such as that required to clean windows should be avoided, and shifting furniture is forbidden unless it is on easy running castors. Digging and heavier gardening tasks should be delegated. The reasons for these precautions must be explained to the patient.

RESULTS OF TOTAL ELBOW REPLACEMENT

Relief of pain is almost universal. Improvement in range of movement is related to the pre-operative condition of the joint. If restricted movement was due to pain, mobility is greatly improved by surgery, but if the joint was stiff, improved motion is less significant. Recent reviews of both the Souter-Strathclyde and Wadsworth prostheses demonstrated that functional flexion, adequate extension, good pronation and supination were restored (Burt *et al.*, unpublished review).

Since rheumatoid patients have multiple joint involvement, the general rule for upper limb surgery is to work from proximal to distal joints (see Chapter 1) for best functional ability. A review of patients who had replacements of both shoulder and elbow joints in the same arm (Friedman and Ewald, 1987) revealed that 75% of them obtained more functional benefit from the elbow arthroplasty than from the shoulder surgery. One conclusion drawn was that if one joint was more painful and immobile than the other, the worse joint should be replaced first.

Early post-operative complications, such as transient ulnar nerve palsy, are usually successfully overcome. The longer term complications which have occurred with hinge prostheses include loosening in a significant number of cases (Morrey, 1985). The incidence of humeral loosening is much higher than that of the ulnar component (Gschwend *et al.*, 1988). Later instability may occur as a result of wearing of the articulation device (Morrey, 1985). These same causes of failure are listed by Souter (1987). Deep infection is also possible. Clearly there have to be revision procedures and salvage operations to deal with these failures.

REVISION OF TOTAL ELBOW REPLACEMENT

The aim with elbow arthroplasty is to remove the minimum of bone stock at the time of primary surgery, so that revision is facilitated should it become necessary. Preservation of the humeral condyles is important, partly for stability and also because the flexor and extensor tendons are attached to them.

Indications for revision of total elbow replacement are loosening of either component, bone fracture due to resorption of the bone as a result of loosening, instability, recurrent dislocation or deep infection. If the coupling mechanism fails in a hinge prosthesis, only the coupling mechanism needs revision.

Removal of the prosthesis tends to be difficult, as the bone cortex may be damaged during removal of the cement and a fracture may occur. If a second arthroplasty is to be inserted, a different type of implant is used. The range of movement after revision surgery has been found to be almost identical to that obtained after primary surgery (Morrey, 1985).

If bone stock is inadequate or if deep infection has occurred, revision may be impossible. In the case of infection, the usual procedure of removal of all foreign material, wound closure and insertion of suction drains until swabs prove negative and soft tissues have healed is carried out. Then salvage surgery may be performed, possibly in the form of interpositional arthroplasty.

Interpositional arthroplasty may occasionally be used in the treatment of the younger post-traumatic arthritis patient. The ends of the humerus, ulna and radius are excised, contoured to facilitate the pivoting of the ulna against the humerus, and soft tissue interposed between the bony surfaces (Wright and Steward, 1985). The patient must be motivated to co-operate fully in the rehabilitation programme. Results of these interpositional arthroplasties are generally good, giving pain relief and reasonable elbow flexion.

Simple excision of the radial head is still occasionally indicated. It relieves pain but interferes with the other structures within the joint and may therefore cause secondary problems. Resection arthroplasty, in which the ends of humerus, radius and ulna are resected, leaving a flail arm, is carried out only to eradicate an intractable joint infection. Elbow arthrodesis is also unacceptable, as there is no optimum position in which to fuse the joint.

Elbow fractures are particularly disabling and are prone to complications such as damage to the brachial artery and the median and ulna nerves. They are not normally treated on the cold (elective) orthopaedic ward, and it is not within the scope of this book to discuss fractures and dislocations of the elbow.

REMEDIAL OCCUPATIONAL THERAPY

Resumption of activities of daily living as a gradual process normally provides all the 'occupational therapy' a patient with rheumatoid arthritis needs. In the case of the younger post-trauma patient, occupational therapy may be prescribed as an adjunct to physiotherapy. Aims and objectives are then similar to those following shoulder replacement.

Normal range of movement for the elbow is flexion-extension 0–150°, 80° each for pronation and supination. The most useful arcs of movement are 30–130° of flexion and 50° each of pronation and supination. Provided these measurements can be attained, it is unnecessary to push for a greater range than this, and it may even be contra-indicated. Extension lag is usual following elbow surgery, and full extension is not essential for most activities.

Sample treatment programme

To obtain the correct movement of flexion and extension the work must be placed directly in front of the patient and close to him.

1. Rest the forearm on a skateboard, push to and fro on a level surface.

2. Polish wood with a to and fro action.
3. Knead and roll soft dough.
4. Play various hand games on a large board.
5. Sand a board with to and fro action; increase resistance by using coarser sandpaper.
6. As (3) and (4) but using dough of stiffer consistency and games with heavier pieces.
7. Build towers with discs.
8. Weave with a long shuttle; macrame knotting.
9. Use of guillotine. Increase resistance by cutting more sheets of paper at a time.
10. Stool seating.

Simultaneously, a programme to obtain pronation and supination requires that the patient's elbow is held close to his body, flexed to 90° and the work placed directly in front of him:

1. Use the wire maze game.
2. Twist a baton, with elbows flexed, holding baton with hands close together.
3. Use of computer game with mercury activation switch attached to wristband.
4. Build towers of discs, picking up disc with forearm pronated and putting it down with forearm supinated.
5. Use of Meccano.
6. Table football.

The activities should be carried out for periods of 5–10 minutes, preferably daily for four sessions per day. Throughout, care must be taken to avoid passive, forced or jerky movement at the joint. Pronation is necessary for placing objects on a horizontal surface, so many activities achieve this movement. Supination may be slower to recover, and compensatory movement is lacking. Possibly the most important task requiring supination is holding out the hand for change. It therefore needs to be worked at!

REFERENCES

Friedman, R.J. and Ewald, F.C. (1987) Arthroplasty of the ipsilateral shoulder and elbow in patients who have rheumatoid arthritis, *Journal of Bone and Joint Surgery,* **69-A**, no. 5, 661–6.

Gschwend, N., Loehr, J., Ivosevic-Radovanovic, D., Scheier, H. and Munzinger, U. (1988) Semi-constrained elbow prostheses with special reference to the GSB III prosthesis, *Clinical Orthopaedics and Related Research,* **232**, 104–11.

Morrey, B.F. (1985) Revision joint replacement, in B.F. Morrey (ed.) *The Elbow and Its Disorders*, W.B. Saunders, Philadelphia.

Souter, W.A. (1987) Surgical management of rheumatoid arthritis, in S.P.F. Hughes, M.K. Benson and C. Colton (eds.) *Orthopaedics: The principles and practice of musculoskeletal surgery*, Churchill Livingstone, Edinburgh.

Wright, P.E. and Steward, M.J. (1985) Fascial arthroplasty of the elbow, in B.F. Morrey (ed.) *The Elbow and Its Disorders*, W.B. Saunders, Philadelphia.

FURTHER READING

Burt, A., Burger, T. and Gwilliam, L. *Review of Patients having had Elbow Replacement at Wrightington Hospital, Wigan*, unpublished paper.

Figgie, M.P., Inglis, A.E., Mow, C.S., Wolfe, S.W., Sculco, T.P. and Figgie III, H.E. (1990) Results of reconstruction for failed total elbow arthroplasty, *Clinical Orthopaedics and Related Research*, **253**, 123–32.

Figgie III, H.E., Inglis, A.E., Ranawat, C.S. and Rosenberg, G.M. (1987) Results of total elbow arthroplasty as a salvage procedure for failed elbow reconstructive operations, *Clinical Orthopaedics and Related Research*, **219**, 185–93.

Ljung, P., Lidgren, L. and Rydholm, U. (1989) Failure of the Wadsworth elbow, *Acta Orthop Scand*, **6**, no. 3, 254–7.

London, J. (1985) Custom arthroplasty and hemiarthroplasty of the elbow, in B.F. Morrey (ed.) *The Elbow and Its Disorders*, W.B. Saunders, Philadelphia.

Madsen, F., Gudmundson, G.H., Sojbjerg, J.O. and Snappen, O. (1989) The Pritchard Mark II elbow prosthesis in rheumatoid arthritis, *Acta Orthop Scand*, **60**, no. 3, 249–53.

Mills, D. and Fraser, C. (1989) *Therapeutic Activities for the Upper Limb*, Winslow Press, Bicester.

Morrey, B.F. and Bryan R.S. (1985) Total joint replacement, in B.F. Morrey (ed.) *The Elbow and Its Disorders*, W.B. Saunders, Philadelphia.

Norkin, C. and Levangie, P. (1989) *Joint Structure and Function: A comprehensive analysis*, F.A. Davis, Philadelphia.

Sjoden, G.O.J., Blomgren, G.G.A. and Lindgren, J.U. (1985) The Souter total elbow replacement in rheumatoid arthritis, *Scandinavian Journal of Rheumatology*, **1**, 219–22.

Trancik, T., Wilde, A.H. and Borden, L.S. (1987) Capitellocondylar total elbow arthroplasty, *Clinical Orthopaedics and Related Research*, **223**, 175–80.

Trombly, C. (1983) *Occupational Therapy for Physical Dysfunction*, Williams and Wilkins, Baltimore.

Turner, A. (1981) *The Practice of Occupational Therapy: An introduction to the treatment of physical dysfunction*, Churchill Livingstone, Edinburgh.

9

The hand

Several complete volumes have been written on the subject of hand rehabilitation and it is not within the scope of this book to cover the topic in any detail. However, the occupational therapist working on the orthopaedic ward must be competent to handle those conditions she may encounter. These include surgery for the rheumatoid hand, tendon injuries, trauma which presents a continuing problem, post-traumatic arthritis and congenital abnormalities.

VERSATILITY OF THE HAND

The hand has multiple functions:

* infinitely fine to powerful movement, including prehensile action;
* used in nearly all activities of daily living;
* major organ of sensation;
* used in self-protection;
* gentle or violent tactile communication;
* gesticulation during speech;
* communication with the deaf;
* the 'eye' of the visually handicapped.

ARCHITECTURE OF THE HAND

The hand is a complex organ. Many individual movements are difficult to isolate, so any impairment will affect total function. The bony structure of the hand forms the foundation for its function, and is based on a series of arches. The transverse arches are first, the arch formed by the carpal bones, and second, the arch formed by the metacarpal heads, this latter being very flexible. The longitudinal arch is formed by the metacarpal and phalangeal bones and is also very adaptable. The oblique arch is formed by the thumb in abduction and opposition to the little finger. The stable element in the arched hand is maintained by the shafts of the second and third metacarpal bones (Figure 9.1a).

When at rest, the normal hand maintains all these arches, with all the muscles relaxed and in a balanced state. The metacarpophalangeal (MCP) joint of the

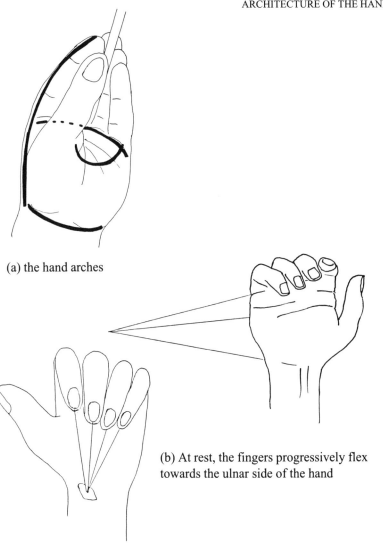

(a) the hand arches

(b) At rest, the fingers progressively flex towards the ulnar side of the hand

(c) In flexion, the fingertips converge on the scaphoid

Figure 9.1 Architecture of the hand

index finger is flexed at approximately 25°, the proximal interphalangeal (PIP) joint flexed at approximately 45°, and the distal interphalangeal (DIP) joint flexed at approximately 15°, with the thumb anterior to the phalanges of the index finger. The palm is hollowed and the fingers progressively flexed, with the index finger straightest and the little finger most flexed (Figure 9. 1b). The fingertips converge towards the scaphoid bone (Figure 9. 1c).

HAND ASSESSMENT

The surgeon may require an occupational therapy assessment of the hand of a patient he is considering for surgery, to enable him to decide on the most appropriate procedure. The purpose of hand assessment is, therefore, to document deformity, hypo-aesthesia, grip and function. Repeated hand assessments gauge improvement and recovery or record deterioration. They are often performed together with a physiotherapy assessment.

At the outset it is essential to read the case notes, to learn the history, definitive diagnosis and reason for performing the assessment. At the initial interview with the patient, a brief explanation of the procedure helps to allay anxiety. Hand dominance must be established. Details of the patient's family role, occupation and leisure interests demonstrate the uses to which he puts his hands. The patient should be asked which are his problem areas in order of severity, to assist in later decision-making regarding action or order of surgery.

On examination, the shoulders and elbows should be checked for limitation in movement. The affected and normal hands are compared. Any differences are noted as to the position of the hand at rest, skin colour, texture and sweating, scars, oedema, muscle wasting, contractures or other deformity and condition of the nails. Palpation of the affected hand provides information as to the skin condition, subluxed joints, boggy areas due to synovitis, tender areas and scars with fibrosis.

If the hand is painful, the patient should be asked to describe the pain, some adjectives being suggested, such as severe pain, discomfort, continual, intermittent, aching, throbbing, burning, tingling, stabbing, etc. He should be asked if anything appears to trigger the pain, or if anything relieves it. A visual analogue may help him describe the pain. This is scaled from 0 to 10, the patient making a subjective rating of his pain on the line, thus:

Painfree	0 1 2 3 4 5 6 7 8 9 10	The worst pain imaginable

Observation of how the patient uses his hand provides additional information. As the hand is also an organ of communication, the patient may hide the hand due to embarrassment.

If the physiotherapist has measured range of joint movement, it is unnecessary for the occupational therapist to duplicate this. If it falls to the occupational therapist to measure joint range, the goniometer is the most usual instrument to use (Figure 9.2). The wrist is measured along the shafts of the ulna and fifth

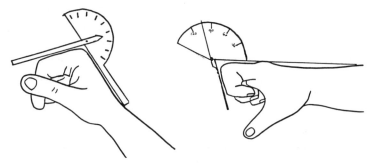

Figure 9.2 Measurement of MCP (left) and PIP (right) joint flexion using goniometers

metacarpal, with the ulnar styloid as the axis. The MCP joints are measured individually, over the shafts of the metacarpal bones and the proximal phalanges, over the dorsum of the joint. The IP joints are measured over the adjacent phalanges and over the dorsum of the IP joints, with the MCP joints extended in order to measure the DIP joints properly, as they normally flex right into the palm. The carpometacarpal joint of the thumb is measured along the shafts of the first and second metacarpals (Figure 9.3). The MCP joint of the thumb is measured along the shafts of the first metacarpal and the proximal phalanx, over

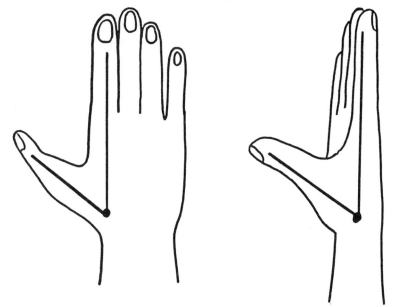

Figure 9.3 Positions for measurement of radial (left) and palmar (right) abduction of the thumb

the dorsum of the joint with the thumb abducted. The IP joint of the thumb is measured along the shafts of the proximal phalanges, over the dorsum of the joint. If oedema is present, the goniometer should be held along the mid shafts of the bones instead of over the dorsum. Where there is significant discrepancy between active and passive range, both figures should be recorded. Joint measurements of the normal hand should also be recorded for comparison. Normal ranges of joint movement in the hand are:

- wrist flexion 70–80°, extension 70–75°;
- radial deviation at the wrist 20°, ulnar deviation 20°;
- pronation 0–80°, supination 0–80°;
- MCP joints 0–90° flexion, PIP joints 0–100° flexion, DIP joints 0–80° flexion;
- thumb carpometacarpal extension 15–45°, abduction 0–70°;
- thumb MCP joint 0–50° flexion;
- thumb IP joint 0–80° flexion.

Hyperextension of a finger joint is recorded as a minus number, extension as zero, extension lag as a plus number. The range of movement is therefore recorded as, for example:

$$\frac{\text{extension}}{\text{flexion}} = \frac{10}{75} \text{ and } \frac{15}{70}$$

The total active flexion of one finger is 175°.

Pronation and supination are measured starting with the forearm and hand placed in the 'thumbs up' position. Excursion movements may be measured with a ruler (Figure 9.4). In abduction the distance between the fingertips can

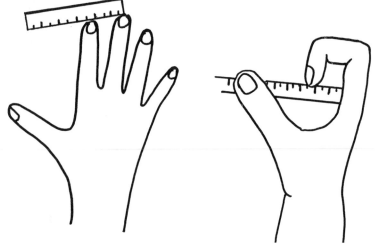

Figure 9.4 Measurement of finger abduction (left) and total finger flexion (right) using a ruler

be measured. If opposition is incomplete, the distance between the thumb tip and the base of each finger is measured. Total finger flexion can be measured at right angles from the transverse palmar crease to the tips of the fingers (normal registers zero). Extension lag of the MCP and IP joints may be measured in this way, with the hand placed on the table in supination. Total span is also measured with a ruler.

Odstock tracings are a recognized method of recording joint range, especially suitable for rheumatoid patients. Soldering wire covered in flexible plastic tubing is used to follow the dorsal aspect of each digit at its maximum range of flexion and extension, then tracing along the wire to record the reading on a chart. The joint positions must be marked (Figure 9.5). To do this the patient sits with the elbow supported on a table, with the wrist in neutral or slight extension. The flexion tracing is superimposed on the extension tracing, using the proximal phalanx as the baseline. Subsequent recordings are traced in a different colour, and each colour code dated.

Hand tracings are a useful method of recording abduction of the MCP joints, ulnar deviation, thumb extension, and apparent shortening due to subluxation or flexion deformity. It involves tracing around the patient's spread hand, marking the joint positions. Again, subsequent tracings are in a different colour and the colour code dated.

Any oedema is most accurately measured by water displacement methods, plunging the hand in a tank with graduations marked on the inner walls. Jewellers' ring measures may also be used to measure oedema in the fingers.

Key baseline, normal extension — — — —
     flexion, first reading
     flexion, later reading

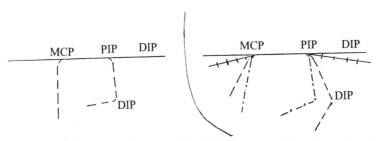

Figure 9.5 Odstock tracings. On the left, the normal hand. On the right, demonstrating improved flexion following surgery

If there is not a concurrent assessment by the physiotherapist, the patient's muscle power should be graded according to the Medical Research Council's Oxford Scale (Adams and Hamblen, 1990), comparing the normal against the affected side. The gradings are as follows:

0—No contraction
1—A flicker
2—Active movement through full range with gravity eliminated
3—Active movement through full range against gravity
4—Active movement through full range with some resistance
5—Normal muscle strength as compared with unaffected side.

Normal grip strength varies greatly from one person to another. Therefore, comparison has to be made between the normal and affected hand. A sphygmomanometer will record a low reading. Five readings should be taken, with a short rest between them. Repetitive measurements are important in distinguishing the malingering patient. Each measurement should be taken by the same therapist in the same way, using the same machine.

Pinch grip may also be recorded using a sphygmomanometer, measuring pinch between thumb and each finger in turn. If the patient is only able to use lateral pinch or three-point pinch this should be recorded as such.

Sensation assessment is performed after nerve damage. The patient is told what to expect. His hand is cradled either in a bead cushion or on a bed of putty, which restricts extraneous movements which may distort results (Moran, 1986). The patient's eyes are closed or his vision blocked by some means. For testing this condition, a hard blunt object is used to test static or moving touch. The two-point discrimination test may be used, with the aid of a paper clip used as a caliper. With the points well apart, the patient's fingers are gently touched longitudinally on the pulps or the whole palmar surface. The patient is asked whether he feels one or two points, administered at random, with the points progressively brought closer together. However, two-point discrimination is a judgement not a primary sensation, and depends in part on the patient's intelligence (Wynn Parry, 1981).

Testing for temperature sensation may be carried out using a cold and a warmed teaspoon. The areas of lost or abnormal sensation should be recorded on a basic hand drawing. Stereognosis tests may be used, with common objects being identified by feel, offering the largest objects to identify first. Pairing objects by the sense of touch is an alternative method.

Proprioception, or joint position sense, may be affected in high median and radial nerve lesions. It is tested by holding the patient's finger on both sides, then moving it slightly in flexion or extension and asking the patient to identify the movement made. The localization test was devised by Wynn Parry (1981). For this, the therapist touches a point on the patient's hand, moving her finger slightly to prevent adaptation of the nerve endings. The patient is asked to open his eyes and point to the area where he was touched. Two pictures are used to record results, one to record where the therapist touched the patient, the other to record where the patient thought he was touched, and the two compared.

The Tinel test documents the level of recovery of a nerve after injury, which grows from proximal to distal at the rate of 1 mm per day. The occupational therapist taps along the course of the affected nerve, from the distal point to the proximal, and the patient will experience pins and needles at the site of nerve regeneration.

During the functional assessment, the various types of grip are tested. The most frequently used grip is the precision grip in its three forms: tip to tip or pulp to pulp between thumb and index finger, lateral (key) pinch in which the pad of the thumb is held against the lateral surface of the index finger, and tripod (chuck or three-point pinch) in which the thumb, index and middle finger converge to hold an object. Interdigital pinch is effective adduction between the index and middle fingers.

Power grip is used to wield tools strongly, with the tool held diagonally across the palm, the fingers and thumb flexed around it and the wrist in ulnar deviation. The MCP joints are in ulnar deviation, and the smaller the tool and the more tightly it is grasped, the greater the degree of ulnar deviation. If the ring and little fingers are weak, this grasp will be ineffective. Sustained grasp is maintained by the wrist flexors.

Cylinder grip involves opening the hand so that the thumb and fingers form a 'C' around an object, then the muscles contract to hold it. It depends on the integrity of all the digits, the interossei and the web space and efficiency of the thumb muscles.

Span grip depends on the hand arches and demands that all digits are extended and abducted first, then the distal phalanges flex to hold the disc.

Ball grip depends on the efficiency of the thenar and hypothenar muscles, and the functioning of the hand arches.

In hook grip, the hand arches are flattened and the fingers flexed at the PIP joints.

Plate grip involves strong opposition of the thumb and flexion of the MCP joints, with extension of the IP joints and a stable wrist.

The types of grip may be assessed as follows:

- Pinch grip: picking up a pin (fine) and a pencil.
- Lateral pinch: picking up and holding a Yale type key.
- Tripod grip: writing with pen or pencil.
- Interdigital pinch: holding a cigarette between the fingers.
- Power grip: holding and effectively using a hammer.
- Cylinder grip: picking up a tumbler of water.

- Span grip: opening a jar with a screw top or a pull-off lid.
- Ball grip: holding different sized balls.
- Hook grip: carrying a bag.
- Plate grip: holding a plate level.
- Pronation and supination: pouring water from one glass to another and back again.

In all the above, it is important to watch for trick movements.

Dexterity and co-ordination are tested by asking the patient to perform a number of common tasks: using a pair of scissors, striking a match, opening and closing a safety pin, fastening an open-ended zip, fastening a wrist watch, handling change in a purse or pocket, threading a needle, signing their name, etc. Any deviation from the normal action in performing these activities is recorded.

Finally, independence in the functions of daily living should be assessed. It is more relevant to first ask the patient what his difficulties are, to ensure that the assessment is more appropriate to his needs. The Odstock Hospital Hand Function Chart takes this a step further, by asking the patient to select from the chart the tasks that are relevant to him, and to grade the ease with which the tasks are performed, as easy, fair, difficult or impossible. The patient and therapist then discuss why these tasks present problems, choosing from a list of reasons which include pain, weakness, thumb problems, MCP joint problems, IP joint problems, wrist or any other joint problems, tendon problems, sensory problems, etc. When the reasons are totalled, the reasons for dysfunction become clear and the analysis is especially helpful if the assessment is to be followed by a period of remedial treatment. (N.B: A patient with rheumatoid arthritis may have grossly deformed hands, yet have relatively good function as compared with another whose hands are minimally deformed but more painful.)

When compiling the hand assessment report, it is convenient to use standard forms. A national standard assessment form is the ideal, but the assessment system should at least be the same across all hospitals in the same group. A sub-committee of the British Orthopaedic Association, all members of the British Society for Surgery of the Hand, met with a view to recommending a design for an assessment form for routine use in Accident and Emergency departments and hand clinics (Robins, 1986). They recognized that no chart could cover all hand conditions but concluded that charts should be simple and consistent in design and flexible in application. The requirements for Accident and Emergency hand charts are distinct from those for specialist hand clinics. For the latter, separate charts are required, any or all of which may be used for one assessment. They include:

- range of movement chart, recording active and passive readings, with space for Odstock tracings;
- sensory chart, with basic hand illustration;

- functional assessment chart.

The chart for use in Accident and Emergency departments includes recording in diagrammatic form scars, tissue damage, sensory loss, etc. and may also be helpful to use with orthopaedic patients.

The combined charts provide the basis for a treatment plan, and may be useful at a later date if needed in medico-legal claims. They are available in A4 pads from Pilgrim's Press (address in appendix) and it is hoped that they will become routinely used.

Hand assessment with a young child

Provided he is of average intelligence, a child can be assessed by the same procedure as an adult from the age of four to five years. With a younger child, it is necessary to provide a box of suitable toys and guide the child through experimentation with them, closely observing his handling of them. It is a time-consuming process. It is very important that the room is quiet with no distractions, so that concentration is enhanced. The occupational therapist must also be aware of the ages at which different aspects of hand function develop.

Basically the same pattern is followed as for adults, but the functional assessment of grip plays a larger part and this may be assessed by observing activities such as the following:

- Pinch grip: threading large beads on a string, picking up a crayon.
- Lateral pinch: picking up a book or pieces of a wooden jigsaw puzzle.
- Tripod grip: scribbling with a crayon.
- Interdigital pinch: squeezing plasticine between the fingers.
- Power grip: playing with a toy hammer and matrix.
- Cylinder grip: holding appropriate kind of mug of milk or fruit juice.
- Span grip: undoing a screw top or pull-off top of a jar of sweets.
- Ball grip: playing ball using balls of different sizes.
- Hook grip: carrying a toy suitcase.
- Plate grip: offering a biscuit on a plate to parent.
- Pronation and supination: playing with Russian dolls or similar toy, un-screwing successive barrels to find small doll in the centre.
- Co-ordination: use of paper-cutting scissors, undoing a small parcel, dress-ing a doll or playing with construction toys.

REHABILITATIVE TREATMENT OF THE HAND

Referrals for specific treatment will vary according to the specialization of the unit in question. The most likely requests will be for splinting following surgery for rheumatoid arthritis, rehabilitation after reconstruction surgery, trauma, tendon surgery and surgical correction of congenital deformity.

Fibrosis can be minimized by controlled mobilization initiated early, otherwise scar tissue contracts and the joint stiffens. Once the wound has healed, remodelling continues for up to a year, while the scar tissue develops the strength and shaping to allow proper function. During this time, passive and active exercises and splinting will assist the remodelling process. The splint may be static or dynamic, intermittent or constant.

Patients whose hands require elective orthopaedic or plastic surgery arrive at this stage for various reasons. Functional loss may be due to pain which has not been adequately controlled, so that the hand has been overprotected. Oedema after injury or surgery is reduced by elevation and if this precaution is neglected, fibrosis occurs.

Stiff joints may result from severe pain, fibrosis, soft tissue contractures and adhesions, damaged blood vessels causing ischaemia, nerve lesions leading to paralysis, fractures near the joint, or to overlong immobilization. Function is of paramount importance and a stiff joint may be more functional than a flail one. Similarly, a muscle that is slightly contracted may have a useful tenodesis effect.

The principle of tenodesis action is that as the proximal joint is moved in one direction, the distal joint moves passively in the opposite direction. For example, in a radial nerve lesion flexion is present at the wrist and fingers but extension is absent, so a wrist extension splint may produce finger flexion. Patients with tetraplegia can sometimes make use of this passive grasp.

In addition to the motor deficiencies, sensory changes occur if nerves are damaged. Nerve injury will cause hypo-aesthesia, changing through hyperaesthesia as regeneration occurs. Hyperpathia is an exaggerated painful response to touch, which can follow a nerve lesion, and such a condition may be treated by the implantation of neurostimulators as described in Chapter 11, or nerve block may be administered by the anaesthetist.

Aims of rehabilitative occupational therapy

Once pain and oedema are under control, the broad aims are to:

1. improve range of movement;
2. improve muscle power;
3. restore function;
4. re-educate sensation, including pain relief;
5. attend to socio-economic and psychological needs.

Documentation of deformity, range of movement and sensation, as already described, is essential.

The physiotherapist and occupational therapist must liaise closely, although the physiotherapist usually works with the patient first. Early intensive treatment is believed to be more beneficial than a treatment plan spread more thinly over a long period. It is important to explain the treatment to the patient early.

The patient should be placed in the optimum position for the activity in question. This may be sitting or standing, and the work must be at the correct height and angle to obtain the required movement. The patient is less likely to use trick movements if he is seated. The patient with an oedematous hand must work with the hand in elevation to reduce the swelling. Work may be placed on a Varitable, on adjustable shelving or an easel, or placed vertically on the wall to achieve this.

Progression of treatment

As with all remedial treatment, progression is through passive, assisted, active and resisted activities, working from gross through to fine movements. While the physiotherapist gives passive exercise, the occupational therapist may not become involved until the patient is capable of assisted movement. Use of pulleys and suspension slings or a limb balancer may be used with various activities. Bilateral activities are to be preferred early in treatment, as this provides rhythm, facilitates a better pattern of movement and prevents neglect of the affected hand. Cord knotting and weaving are useful activities. If possible, an activity related to the patient's interests and skills should be chosen.

Some activities for gross hand movement

Exercises in warm water and kneading and rolling of theraplast, sanding, use of a guillotine, printing machine, Nomeq 'hand grab', span games, Russian dolls, table football and solitaire using large pegs.

Some activities for medium hand movement

Varnishing small woodwork items, paper folding, sorting nuts and bolts, use of scissors, weaving, threading large beads, draughts, dominoes, rolling crepe bandages, various adaptations of solitaire, use of clothes pegs.

Some activities for fine hand movement

Origami, writing, drawing, composing type, macrame with fine twine, use of tweezers, solitaire with map pins, drawing pins and dress pins, sewing, making a chain with paper clips, untying string with a pin.

Remedial games

Games are readily adaptable for all types of hand exercise. Solitaire pieces can be chunky, weighted, magnetic or attached to the board with velcro to provide resistance. By placing the board in different positions, further movements can be obtained. The patient is instructed in the method of picking up the pegs in the manner which gives the required movement, and is watched carefully to ensure that the desired action is obtained. Solitaire is useful in that it does not need another player. Many other games are suitable for adaptation, but require a partner.

Simple but effective treatment media can be improvised from items such as rubber bands on a nail board, cat's cradle games, marbles, rice and clothes pegs. At the other end of the spectrum, computer games, word processors, typewriters or pianos provide effective hand exercise.

Grasp

This is obtained by the use of rubber syringe bulbs for games such as puff football, and squeezing water from one flask to another, using gross grasp. It may also be obtained by the use of a large firm sponge, using it to transfer the water from one bowl to another.

Wrist flexion and extension

This action is achieved with the use of a 'ski jump' board, to which the arm is fastened proximal to the wrist, with the hand over the end of the board. The object is to pick up shapes by flexing the wrist and then extend the wrist to 'post' the shapes through a postbox in front of the 'ski jump' (Figure 9.6). There are variations on this theme (Figure 9.7). Table tennis using the back of the hand, either with a bat strapped onto the hand or wearing a stiff glove, obtains flexion and extension of the wrist.

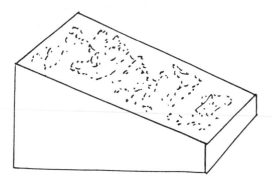

Figure 9.6 Apparatus to assist with hand and wrist rehabilitation, reduce oedema etc. The wooden box is covered with carpet for comfort. The forearm is positioned with the wrist at the higher end, to facilitate flexion or extension

118

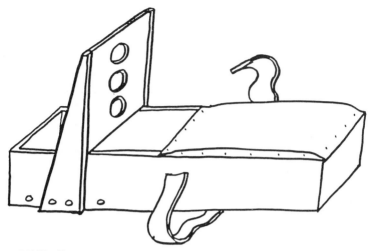

Figure 9.7 Similar apparatus with adjustable upright to encourage wrist flexion in picking up objects, and extension in "posting" them through holes in upright

MCP flexion and extension

Games using rubber syringe bulbs are useful here too, but ensuring that the IP joints are straight. The same applies to the activity with a sponge to transfer water from one bowl to another. Solitaire may be played using tongs or clothes pegs to move the pieces, keeping the IP joints straight. Rubber bands may be stretched over a nail board to play the 'boxes' game, and cat's cradle, rolling theraplast or bandages, walking the fingers up a small ladder placed close to the patient and games involving flicking a ball up a slope are all useful activities.

IP flexion and extension

The bulb syringe games are again suitable, using gross grasp, and the same applies to the sponge squeezing activity. The rubber band 'boxes' game, cat's cradle, bandage rolling, flicking games and tweezer games are suitable. With tweezers, a blocker must be used to prevent the MCP joints compensating. Putty pinch and solitaire using tongs and clothes pegs to pick up the pieces are also useful.

Pinch grip

The bulb syringe games and the sponge squeezing activity are suitable, using the thumb with either the index finger alone or with the index and middle fingers. Tweezers, putty pinch, threading beads and solitaire using pins, tongs or clothes pegs to move the pieces may be tried. Darts uses tripod grip.

Finger abduction and adduction

Solitaire may be used, picking up the pieces between the index and middle fingers, and a tug-of-war game can be played with a piece of paper held between these same two fingers. Putty may be squeezed between all the fingers.

Ingenious minds will invent other ways of obtaining movements required, and the section on occupational therapy in the work by Wynn Parry (1981) gives many ideas. Coiled pottery, breadmaking and other baking activities provide much excellent hand exercise. Use of the FEPS (flexion, extension, pronation and supination) adaptor with printing and use of the wire twisting machine provide a range of useful remedial actions, particularly if full use is made of the different handle attachments.

If staff time is limited, the patient may be given a supplementary programme to follow at home, with suggested activities and a timetable. He must keep a record of his self-treatments and the occupational therapist must monitor the programme.

Sensory re-education

This aspect of remedial treatment is mainly associated with nerve lesions. The selected patient must be well-motivated, intelligent, and should already have return of protective sensation and touch perception in the fingertips (Moran, 1986). The rationale behind sensory re-education is that the patient with sensory impairment can use learning mechanisms to make the most of hand function, in spite of the nerve fibres being somewhat disorganized as compared with the pre-morbid state. The brain gradually responds more efficiently to the reduced sensation, and as it does so, motor function also improves. The sensory stimulation must be carried out early, once the above criteria can be met.

The patient is blindfolded, then given some form of sensory stimulus such as an everyday object to hold, which he is asked to identify. If he is correct, he is told so, but if incorrect he is shown the object, to link the experience of vision with the sense of touch. Later in the session, the process is repeated so that he integrates the visual memory with the present experience. The sessions should be short and frequent, the maximum time being 15 minutes up to three times daily (Moran and Callahan, 1986).

Localization training is also carried out. Blindfolded, the patient is touched on the hand. With the blindfold removed, he is asked to point to the spot where he was touched. If incorrect, the stimulus is repeated while he watches. He then closes his eyes and concentrates while the stimulus is repeated. This concentration, feedback and repetition are crucial to the re-education programme.

Texture discrimination employs pieces of wood covered with different grades of sandpaper and pieces of different fabric. The patient is asked to feel two blocks and say whether they are the same or different, and as treatment progresses, the two grades become more alike. Wooden blocks can have letters stuck on them made of velcro hooks or coarse to medium sandpaper, and the patient asked to identify the letter. All these exercises are carried out with the eyes closed or the vision blocked.

If motor function is adequate, the patient may be blindfolded, then asked to pick objects out of a bowl of rice, starting with large items working towards smaller. Plastic alphabet letters may be used in a similar manner. Everyday objects may be put into a closed bag, and the patient asked to identify them by feel. At first objects are dissimilar but as progress is made, the objects chosen are more alike. While his eyes are closed, the therapist may draw letters on the patient's hand with her finger, and the patient asked to identify them.

The sensory training can be integrated into the motor function programme by drawing the patient's attention to the textures and shape of the objects used. The use of drills, saw, hammer, etc. will cause vibration, which makes a positive contribution to sensation training.

The use of sensory re-training is valuable in the desensitizing of the finger stump following amputation.

HAND SURGERY ON THE ORTHOPAEDIC WARD

As mentioned earlier, the majority of surgery will be for the rheumatoid hand. It may be helpful at this point to look back at Chapter 1 at the general effects of the disease, and specifically at the effects on the hand. The inflammation in the synovium around the carpus affects the capsule and ligaments supporting the joint, and ligaments may become stretched. The palmar and dorsal pull of the muscle tendons becomes unbalanced, the proximal row of carpal bones migrates towards the palmar surface, the distal row of carpals migrates dorsally, and subluxation occurs. The extensor carpi ulnaris tendon may be damaged in the process, and may slip towards the palm and become a flexor. Because the extensor carpi radialis longus and brevis and the flexor carpi radialis are now unopposed, radial deviation of the wrist and ulnar deviation of the MCP joints occur. The elongation of the radial collateral ligaments contributes to the deformity. Palmar subluxation of the MCP joints is also caused by slack ligaments.

Boutonniere deformity is due to the disruption of the extensor mechanism at the PIP joint, resulting in flexion of the PIP joint and hyperextension of the DIP joint. It is difficult to treat. The extensor tendon may be re-attached more proximally but may then cause mallet finger. Activities aim at flexion of the distal joint and extension of the proximal, with the use of a Capener splint (Figure 9.8).

Mallet finger is caused by a ruptured extensor tendon proximal to the distal phalanx, so that this phalanx is flexed by the pull of the flexor digitorum

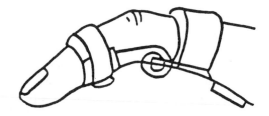

Figure 9.8 Capener splint

profundus tendon, and a portion of bone may be involved. Surgical repair may leave permanent stiffness so treatment is by splinting the DIP joint in extension for six weeks to unite the torn tendon (Hughes, 1989). If the splint is removed during this time, the finger must be supported.

Swan neck deformity is caused by imbalance of the flexor digitorum superficialis causing hyperextension of the lax PIP joint, with secondary flexion of the DIP joint. It may be treated with a small splint to prevent hyperextension of the proximal joint, or by a two-stage flexor tendon graft with a silastic rod.

Synovectomy

Synovectomy is indicated when bone destruction is not advanced but proliferation of synovial tissue is marked. The inflamed synovium surrounding the joint is excised and if the tendons are involved, tenosynovectomy may be performed. Good results are obtained when this operation is performed in the dorsum of the hand, and will slow down the damage which may cause ruptured tendons. The procedure usually has to be repeated, as the benefits rarely persist. A secondary effect of flexor synovitis is carpal tunnel syndrome.

Carpal tunnel syndrome

The median nerve may be compressed at wrist level under the transverse carpal ligament (flexor retinaculum) as it passes in the carpal tunnel with the tendons of the finger flexors and the tendon of flexor pollicis longus. There is first a sensory loss, commonly at night, which may extend into the forearm. Motor weakness of abductor pollicis brevis, opponens pollicis, flexor pollicis brevis and the first and second lumbricals ensues. The patient is inclined to be clumsy and drop things, and complains of burning pain with numbness and then tingling in the thumb and first two fingers and half the ring finger, especially during the night and early morning. Two-point discrimination can be tested in the distribution of the median nerve. Treatment is by splinting and injection of steroid, and if the problem is not resolved, then electromyographic testing before surgical division of the flexor retinaculum. Although the condition is commonly a result of rheumatoid arthritis, it may be due to various causes including Colles' fracture. Usually only one wrist is operated on at a time, even if the condition is bilateral, so that the patient can cope with daily living activities. Unless there are complicating circumstances, the only specific occupational therapy needed may be the provision of a night resting splint with the wrist in no more then 30° of extension. A Futuro splint worn at night decreases symptoms.

WRIST SURGERY

Rheumatoid disease of the wrist joint leads to deformity, pain, instability and loss of function. Osteo-arthritic changes may occur secondary to trauma, when pain may be severe and function impaired. Surgery is indicated in such cases.

In radiocarpal arthritis, where the proximal row of carpal bones is most affected, a proximal row carpectomy may be performed. The wrist is immobilized for four weeks, then range of movement and strengthening exercises commenced, with a protective palmar wrist splint for a further eight weeks or more. The disadvantage of this procedure is that the resulting musculotendinous shortening reduces the strength in the fingers. However, it may allow movement in an otherwise painful wrist. Proximal row carpectomy is normally done at the time of Swanson total wrist replacement.

Total wrist replacement

The most commonly used implant in replacement of the wrist joint is made of silicone rubber which is protected by titanium grommets (Figure 9.9). This implant was designed by Alfred Swanson in the early 1960s and has gone through several stages of evolution. Other types of prosthetic design have been used, including unconstrained metal prostheses with high density polyethylene articulation (e.g. the Meuli), but these are not extensively used so the following discussion will be confined to the Swanson silicone implant.

This implant acts as an inert spacer which is inserted after excision of the proximal row of carpal bones. The implant is inserted into the distal radial medullary cavity, and through the capitate into the third metacarpal, and not cemented. Encapsulation of the implant occurs to hold it in place. An essential part of the surgical procedure is careful re-alignment of tendons and ligaments to balance the wrist joint. Silicone arthroplasty of the wrist joint aims to provide pain relief with some movement. Excessive movement, i.e. greater than 30° of flexion or extension, increases the incidence of fracture of the implant which is then frequently associated with pain, and often necessitates re-operation. This may be revision of the implant or arthrodesis may be chosen.

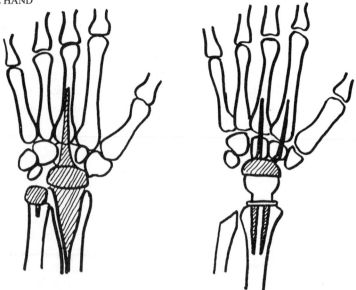

Figure 9.9 Total wrist replacements: Swanson silastic implant on the left. On right, Meuli prosthesis, showing eccentric placement of anchoring stems

Wrist replacement is used almost exclusively for rheumatoid disease. Contra-indications are previous infections of the joint, ruptured wrist extensors or insufficient bone stock. However, patients who do heavy manual work or who use crutches or other walking aids are also unsuitable candidates. Success of the surgery depends on the severity of the disease and musculotendinous balance. The Swanson implant has proved successful in the relief of pain, improvement of function and correction of deformity, with patients expressing satisfaction with the results. In addition, as cement is not used, revision surgery is facilitated.

POST-OPERATIVE CARE

Initial splinting of the wrist in the neutral position is maintained for three weeks. The overall time for immobilization depends on the nature of the patient's disease. Some patients with rheumatoid arthritis have very stiff joints as a result of the disease process, while in others the joints are lax and unstable. Patients with lax, unstable joints need splinting for much longer than those in the first category, so that previously lax structures can shorten.

Early treatment includes routine care of adjacent joints and reduction of swelling. Particular attention is paid to maintaining good excursion of the extensor digitorum tendons, as they are routinely moved outside the extensor retinaculum and are therefore subcutaneous and at risk of adherence to the healing scar if full excursion is not maintained.

After the initial period of immobilization, be it three or six weeks, movement of the wrist joint is commenced. The aim is not to achieve a wide range but to limit the arc of movement to 30° each side of neutral, with 5° radial and 10° ulnar deviation. For most patients this range is not difficult to achieve. Simple wrist exercises followed by normal activity are all that is required to restore function. It is essential to teach the patient joint protection methods so that they do not exceed the stated range of movement, and to guard against rotary strains which may tear the implant.

The maximum weight a patient can lift depends entirely on his own musculature, and it is essential to stress that any weight that cannot be controlled by the wrist muscles must not be attempted. Weightbearing through the joint is prohibited, and any patient whose lifestyle places heavy demands on the implant is a failure of the pre-operative selection process and would be instructed to wear a strong wrist support during heavy activity. The versatility of the hand is aided by the ability of the wrist to place the hand in a variety of positions. It is, therefore, preferable to maintain a mobile wrist, especially in those people whose livelihood depends on this. A wrist arthroplasty will not provide full range of movement, but such a range is not needed for function. Since rheumatoid arthritis tends to affect corresponding bilateral joints, many surgeons choose to arthrodese one joint and replace the other, to obtain maximum function. This, for example, will render a patient independent in the sensitive issue of toilet hygiene, which requires a mobile wrist. This achievement of maximum function is especially important, as other joints will be involved, and the cumulative effect of several impaired joints is very disabling.

Patients with post-traumatic arthritis of the wrist are likely to develop loosening of a wrist prothesis, due to the normality of their other tissues and higher levels of activity. It is, therefore, preferable for these patients to have an arthrodesis instead.

Wrist arthrodesis

This may be used to stabilize the wrist either as a primary operation or as a salvage procedure, for deep infection, prosthetic loosening, musculotendinous imbalance, or in the case of ruptured wrist extensors in the patient with rheumatoid disease. The joint surfaces are excised and fixation achieved by one of the following methods:

- a Steinman pin through the carpus into the radius;
- a Steinman pin into the medullary cavity of the third metacarpal;
- a Rush pin into the base of the third metacarpal, plus a staple across the radiocarpal joint (Figure 9.10).

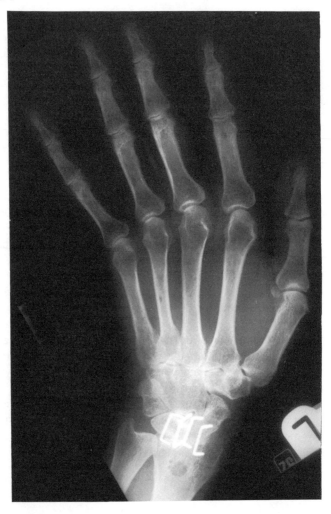

Figure 9.10 Wrist arthrodesis using staples to aid fixation

Occasionally bone grafting is employed to augment the fixation, if bone stock is deficient. Immobilization is maintained for six to 12 weeks after surgery, until bony union.

No remedial occupational therapy is required but the patient may need help in becoming independent in the activities of daily living, with possible provision of tools for living, such as tap turners, jar openers, etc. By the time he has reached this stage, the patient with rheumatoid arthritis may well have many tools already.

MCP JOINT REPLACEMENT

There are other types of semi-constrained MCP implants of metal and plastic but the Swanson silastic implant, or the similar Niebauer reinforced with Dacron, are by far the most popular (Souter, 1987).

Indications for surgery include disorganized MCP joints with severe pain, ulnar drift so great that tripod grip is impossible and which is not correctable by soft tissue surgery, subluxation or dislocation of the joint, radiological evidence of joint destruction, and flexion contractures of the MCP and PIP joints where the palmar skin is macerated (Souter, 1987). MCP joint replacement may be the treatment of choice for a patient with lesser problems but whose life tasks require pinch rather than power grip.

The nature of the MCP joints is somewhat different from that of the wrist and a much wider range of movement is expected. However, the nature of the implant is the same. Excision of the joint surfaces, with synovectomy of the joint, is followed by insertion of an inert flexible spacer into the intramedullary canals of the bones either side of the joint being replaced. This is subsequently surrounded by a synovial-like layer of tissue that provides stability.

The use of these implants has not been without problems. Peimer (1989) believes the most serious fault is the wear-induced debris which occurs in the joint, causing inflammation and secondary bone and joint damage. This is called silicone synovitis. The damage is related to the length of time since implantation, and follow-up surveys of under three years will not demonstrate these problems. These silicone implants should not be used where they will be employed for prolonged, repetitive or forceful work. Souter names the failure to regain power of grasp or pinch grip as a disappointing feature of this surgery. If silicone synovitis occurs, an alternative arthroplasty or joint fusion may be necessary.

Surveys report significant pain relief and an improvement in ulnar deviation. Bieber *et al.* (1986) report improved flexion and extension. Jensen *et al.* (1986) report unchanged range of movement, but a move towards extension, with the hand more open. At the long term evaluation deterioration of the implant has occurred, but one has to remember the progressive nature of rheumatoid disease and balance that fact with any possible deficiencies in the procedure.

Post-operative occupational therapy

The regime most commonly followed is based on that described by Swanson himself (Swanson *et al.*, 1978), early controlled movement being the main principle. Movement wearing a lively outrigger splint is commenced at approximately three to five days post-operatively The splint should support the joints in the neutral position, protect against ulnar deviation, and allow maximum flexion of the joint. Frequent, short periods of exercise are encouraged. Initially it may be necessary to assist the movements and it is always necessary to check that movement is taking place at the level of the MCP joints and not at the PIP joints. If the patient has a tendency to concentrate their movements at the PIP joints, then these joints can be immobilized to concentrate flexion forces towards the MCP joints.

Passive stretching and flexion traction splints for the MCP joints are introduced at three weeks post-operatively. The splint is used for short periods several times a day, and alternated with the outrigger. The outrigger is discarded at approximately six weeks but therapy, both formal and informal, is continued for several months. The expected outcome is a functional arc of flexion and extension at the MCP joints, with a greater flexion range in the ulnar digits and pulp-to-pulp opposition to all digits.

Long term protection of silastic MCP joint replacements is essential and the occupational therapist should ensure that the patient has the necessary knowledge, tools and adaptations to implement joint protection techniques.

Alternative surgery for the MCP joints

A procedure less frequently performed now is simple excision of the metacarpal heads, with or without insertion of interpositional membrane (tendon), or construction of a fascial or ligamentous sling (Souter, 1987).

BASAL THUMB JOINT SILASTIC ARTHROPLASTY

These implants are also of Swanson design, and the criteria for surgery are as for arthroplasty of the MCP joints. The trapezium is excised and part of the trapezoid may be removed to better accommodate the implant, which is then inserted into the intramedullary canal of the thumb metacarpal.

Surveys of surgery on a group of patients who had had these arthroplasties at least 5.5 years previously reported 95% patient satisfaction (Hofammann *et al.*, 1987). By this time a few had considerably deteriorated but results proved that the procedure can relieve pain and improve function over several years. Pinch and grip strength require a stable carpometacarpal joint, and this increases in the majority of cases. Because of later complications, the technique is recommended only for the elderly or the patient whose activity is very limited. Interpositional arthroplasty using tendon is an alternative. The MCP joint of the thumb may be arthrodesed.

Occupational therapy following basal thumb joint arthroplasty

Post-operatively the hand is splinted on the palmar aspect for approximately two weeks. This splint is then replaced by a thumb opponens splint for a further four to six weeks, although surgeons differ in their preference for the type of splint used. After this, gentle active exercise is commenced, while a resting splint may be used at other times. Splinting is discontinued at approximately ten weeks after surgery.

SURGERY INVOLVING TENDONS

Primary tendon repair may be carried out, secondary to trauma. On the cold orthopaedic ward, tendon transfer is the more likely procedure, performed on patients with rheumatoid arthritis or those who have contractures due to neurological conditions. Tendon transfer enables another muscle to perform the function of a damaged or absent one. There are many different transfers available as surgical options.

We have already looked at the effect of rheumatoid disease on synovial joints, and the possibility of tenosynovitis. Rheumatoid nodules may also develop within the tendons. Both these processes interfere with the gliding of the tendons within their sheaths. The extensors of the fingers are particularly vulnerable and may rupture due to erosion or attrition when passing over the ulnar styloid, or due to mechanical stress. The tendons usually snap in a particular order, starting with the little finger, progressing to the ring and then the middle finger, causing the typical dropped finger. Repair is by suturing the distal fragment to the surviving extensors of the adjacent finger or using a palmaris graft. Following extensor tendon repair, the hand should be splinted for four to six weeks, either with the PIP joints immobilized but allowing the DIP joints to flex, or some surgeons prefer full palmar slab splint. The joint is then mobilized, possibly using a dynamic splint to assist in proximal joint extension.

Goniometer measurements are useful for monitoring progress and for giving feedback to patients. Eight weeks after repair, exercise can be more vigorous and some gentle resisted exercise commenced, aimed at useful function. Night extension splints may be required for several more weeks.

The flexor tendons are stronger, and repair within the flexor sheath often results in stiffness. Repair is by suturing the severed ends together, followed by protective splinting. Tendon grafts are used for failed flexor tendon repair. Treatment aims to allow protected movement, and passive movement is delayed until 12 weeks post-operatively. After this period, the aim is for full range of movement followed by developing grip strength, while still allowing full finger extension. A splint such as a Klevier rubber band splint allows protected movement. If the nerve is also damaged, splinting may be required for three weeks before movement is commenced. If heavy activity is appropriate, it must be built up in a graded manner.

Tenolysis

This is the surgical release of adhesions, particularly in the tendon sheath, to allow improved gliding of the tendon. Immediately after surgery, exercise is commenced and a night splint applied. Wearing of this splint alternates with exercise periods for up to six months.

Occupational therapy following tendon surgery

After flexor tendon surgery, any activity which involves picking up objects is therapeutic and various (adapted) hand games may be used, involving light repetitive grip in the early stages. A variety of tool handles should be used to obtain the various types of grip, and the different attachments on the wire twisting machine and the FEPS adaptation are ideal. Handles may need to be lightly padded or covered with a textured material at first. Later a double finger stall may encourage use of the affected digit if recovery is slow. Woodwork and gardening provide excellent gradable activity.

After extensor tendon repair, games or activities involving flicking movements of the fingers, cat's cradle games, and trying to break a match placed over the dorsum of the middle finger and under the distal phalanges of the index and ring fingers are useful.

NERVE INJURIES

As these are usually the result of trauma, relatively few cases will be found on the cold orthopaedic ward. However, Erb's palsy is a brachial plexus lesion caused by a birth injury, usually a breech presentation. In mild cases, slow recovery takes place. In more severe cases, the shoulder is held in adduction and internal rotation and soft tissue contractures may develop and lead to fixed deformity. The mother is taught to put the limb through the full range of movement to prevent this. If fixed deformity does occur, osteotomy, tendon transfer or shoulder arthrodesis may be performed.

Brachial plexus lesions are most often caused by motorcycle accidents, when the shoulder and neck are distracted, causing avulsion of the roots of the brachial plexus. If this occurs the prognosis is very poor, repair being impossible. If the lesion is preganglionic, without avulsion of the nerve roots, the effects are either axonotmesis or neurotmesis. Axonotmesis results in very slow and possibly incomplete recovery, the nerve sheath being intact. Neurotmesis is a complete severence of the nerve, but repair by suture or grafting is possible. Again recovery is only partial, taking two to three years.

Nerve regeneration proceeds at the rate of 1 mm per day. It is important, therefore, that the patient is assessed early, provided with night resting and

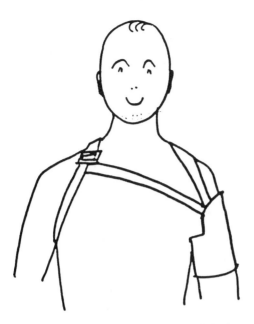

Figure 9.11 Hemi-arm sling, useful for control of the humerus after brachial plexus lesion

working splints, given any necessary training in daily living activities, and an intensive therapy programme for a few weeks. A limb balancer is helpful to support the affected arm. During this period the patient is given a supplementary programme to follow at home, using wide shoulder movements such as polishing, assisting the affected with the good arm. Wearing a Futuro type support splint or a working splint, any kind of activity is beneficial. Sensory assessment and stimulation form part of the treatment plan. The position of the humerus is controlled by a hemi-arm sling, worn under clothing, to prevent shoulder subluxation. The design facilitates positioning without pulling on the back of the neck, and is commercially available (Figure 9.11).

If it is feasible, the patient should return to work as soon as possible, so that he does not get out of the work habit and become increasingly depressed. It is likely that work assessment and resettlement will be necessary.

A flail arm splint is available from Hugh Steeper via the Limb Fitting Centre. It is like the skeleton of an arm prosthesis, and it enables the patient to use his arm during the recovery period. He receives a ten-day training course in use of the prosthesis, and is then encouraged to resume work. Different distal attachments can be fitted to the prosthesis according to need.

Pain is usually severe. It may be relieved by transcutaneous electrical nerve stimulation (TENS) given by the physiotherapist, who also gives the patient an exercise routine to follow at home, and hydrotherapy may also be used. The alternative to the intensive course of treatment is for the patient to attend for treatment two or three times a week for several months, up to two years. Whichever course is adopted, re-assessment will be needed at intervals over the two years. After three years, the muscle fibres become fibrosed and no further motor recovery occurs.

Radial nerve lesions may be caused by axillary pressure or damage at the time of fracture of the humeral shaft. The radial nerve supplies the extensors of the elbow, wrist, fingers and thumb, and the supinator of the forearm. The typical picture is that of dropped wrist. If the patient flexes the wrist fully the MCP and IP joints will extend, and this tenodesis effect may be used at first until recovery occurs. Grasp and release movements are used with a variety of activities and using tools with different shaped handles.

Median nerve lesions most often occur at the wrist joint and the effect has been described under carpal tunnel syndrome. The flat or 'monkey' hand is the typical deformity, with the thumb adducted and the thenar eminence and thumb web atrophied in long-standing cases. Sensory impairment is apparent on the palmar surface of the hand over the thumb, first and second fingers and the radial half of the ring finger. Pronation and wrist flexion are weak and the DIP joints are extended if the lesion is above the wrist. When making a fist, only the ring and little fingers fully flex. The level of muscle involvement depends on the level where the nerve lesion occurred. A thumb splint is required after surgical repair, holding the thumb in abduction and opposition. The median nerve is essential for opposition, tripod and lateral pinch grip.

Ulnar nerve lesions around the elbow or ulnar aspect of the forearm result in the typical claw hand deformity, with the ring and little fingers hyperextended at the MCP joints, the IP joints flexed, hypothenar wasting, and apparent flattening of the arches of the hand. Excursion of the digits is weak, as is the whole hand, due to paralysis of the interossei and adductor pollicis. Most fine movements are absent, and power, span and hook grip are affected. Sensation is lost over the ulnar side of the hand, the little finger and ulnar aspect of the ring finger. If the lesion is at wrist level or distal to the wrist, the short muscles of the hand only are affected, and only the fingers lack sensation. A knuckle duster splint is required to correct hyperextension of the MCP joints and to restore the transverse arch of the hand.

The splints must be worn while the patient works with the hand, and early use is encouraged with all types of lesion. A variety of tools and activities must be employed using repetitive movements, probably padding handles and controls with foam.

If regeneration is not possible, tendon transfer surgery may be employed in order to gain some function.

DUPUYTREN'S CONTRACTURE

Patients with this condition are often admitted for orthopaedic or plastic surgery. The condition is due to thickening of the palmar aponeurosis, commonly with fibrosis and contracture of the ring and little fingers. It may progress to the middle and index fingers or thumb. Surgery involves excision of the affected palmar fascia, with careful preservation of the digital nerves. Occasionally amputation may be indicated. Some patients are left with an open wound after fasciectomy. This is known as the open palm technique.

Post-operatively, exercise of shoulder and elbow helps to maintain good circulation, and at two to three days careful stretching exercises, with gentle flexion, extension and abduction of the fingers and opposition of the thumb, are commenced. Splinting regimes vary but a night splint worn for six months post-operatively may be indicated.

If pain and increasing stiffness and swelling occur, this must be reported to the surgeon immediately, as it may be the onset of reflex sympathetic dystrophy.

REFLEX SYMPATHETIC DYSTROPHY

This term has been suggested as an umbrella phrase for disabilities which have as common signs and symptoms vasomotor instability associated with pain, oedema and skin changes. It includes Sudeck's atrophy and shoulder-hand syndrome. It may occur very soon after soft tissue injury or surgery, Colles' fracture or crush injuries, or may not develop until some weeks after the predisposing cause. It may be due to an exaggerated reaction of the sympathetic nervous system. The earlier signs and symptoms are severe pain in the hand, with oedema, skin colour and temperature changes, excessive sweating and reluctance to move the hand. Later, the skin becomes dry, cold, shiny and blue, the hand stiffens and osteoporosis occurs. Pain is the primary cause, with other changes being secondary, and inactivity becomes the secondary causative factor (Cailliet, 1986).

Prevention is better than cure. After injury or surgery, the hand is elevated to relieve oedema and venous congestion. The joints above and below the affected one should be left free and movement encouraged, while the affected part is comfortably immobilized.

Once the condition has occurred, the pain cycle must be interrupted quickly with analgesics. Unaffected joints must be moved actively and often, and passive movements avoided. Movement should be through the full range and isometric exercises used to reduce oedema and venous congestion. Guanethidine block or TENS may be used to relieve pain.

FINGER AMPUTATION

If this is encountered on the orthopaedic ward it may be as a result of trauma, a tumour, or the last resort in the treatment of Dupuytren's contracture. A crude digit may be moulded and attached to the hand in the same way as an old-fashioned finger stool, in order to maintain movement patterns while engaging in some absorbing activity. This is only practicable when the scar has fully healed. The patient must be encouraged to touch objects. Gentle tapping of the stump helps to desensitize it, so that the patient gains the confidence to use it. This is important because the sensory input lessens the sensation of phantom pain.

CONGENITAL ABNORMALITIES

Congenital abnormalities of the hand are many and varied. The following are those most likely to be admitted for orthopaedic or plastic surgery.

Syndactyly

This implies two or more digits joined together, and appears bilaterally in nearly 50% of cases. The middle and ring finger are most often affected. In simple syndactyly the union is by soft tissue only, while complex syndactyly involves the bone, muscles and blood supply. The aim of surgery is to separate the fingers. A wide web space is necessary to enable the patient to hold a larger object. Timing of surgery is important, depending on the deformity itself and the stage of development of the child. Early surgery is indicated if two digits of disparate length are joined, otherwise secondary deformity in the form of flexion contracture will develop in the longer digit. Surgery prior to starting school is desirable, to prevent teasing and to avoid interrupted schooling later.

Camptodactyly

This is a flexion deformity of the little finger, and may involve the ring and middle fingers, only the PIP joint being affected. Secondary hyperextension of the MCP joint may be present. It is not evident at birth and may not even be noticed until the adolescent growth spurt. Static and dynamic splinting is the treatment of choice, maintained for at least a year. Some authorities recommend night splinting up to skeletal maturity.

Absent thumb

The thumb accounts for 45% of hand function. As children are very adaptable, the child without a thumb usually becomes adept at using his hand, substituting interdigital pinch for handling small objects. In time the web space between the digits widens and some rotation of the index finger occurs, so it becomes more like a thumb. The child still has difficulty in handling larger objects.

Pollicization is the usual procedure for this condition. It fulfils the need to handle larger objects and makes the defect less noticeable and more socially acceptable. Surgery involves the transposition of the index finger and widening the web space. Some modification of the appearance of the new thumb is necessary, because the PIP joint of the index finger simulates the MCP joint of the thumb. Again, surgery is desirable before the child starts school.

Pollicization using a toe to form a thumb may be performed. It is useful where other digits are absent or deformed. Cosmetically the second toe is more acceptable than the great toe and leaves the donor foot with better function and appearance. The epiphyses are intact after the transfer, so the toe/thumb continues to grow with the child.

Radial club hand

This deformity is due to total or partial absence of the radius, usually with an unstable wrist and possible deformity of the radial digits. The condition is frequently bilateral and other congenital deficiencies are often present. The appearance is of a shortened forearm, with the radial side shorter and a prominent ulnar head. The more radius there is, the less the deformity. The ulna is also shortened, and the thumb deformed or absent. The greater the degree of radial deviation and thumb abnormality, the greater is the disability. The ulnar side of the hand is functional, the child becoming accustomed to use the little finger to pick up objects.

The soft tissues are involved, with the superficial radial nerve usually absent below the elbow, while the superficial dorsal branch of the median nerve takes over sensory distribution. This latter nerve is in a vulnerable position during surgery, as it is superficially situated on the radial aspect of the forearm. The radial artery is usually absent, while the median artery takes over its function. Many muscles are fused together, or are abnormal in their origins and insertions.

Children adapt to the disability and become independent in daily living activities, but have to use two hands to perform them.

Treatment depends on the severity of the deformity, functional impairment, age and physical condition of the child, and many need no treatment. Others cannot be helped by surgery. If passive correction is possible, it is maintained by splinting until skeletal maturity. The most commonly used surgical procedure is centralization of the hand over the ulna, to increase function, stabilize the wrist and improve appearance. Surgery is best performed up to the age of three years. A second operation, such as pollicization, may be needed.

Hypoplastic digits

Distraction lengthening techniques may be employed to improve under-developed thumbs and fingers, providing the metacarpals are adequate.

Cleft hand

This is a central defect of the hand, typically V-shaped with a cleft between the metacarpal bones, so the hand is divided into two compartments. It is often combined with syndactyly, and other skeletal abnormalities are common. The atypical cleft hand is U-shaped. The thumb and little finger are present but other digits may be missing or rudimentary.

Surgery for the typical cleft hand deformity is aimed at improving function, with abduction and opposition the main goal. For the atypical cleft hand, the aim is to obtain effective opposition between radial and ulnar sides of the hand.

Cerebral palsy

Orthopaedic surgery can be of real benefit to the cerebral palsy patient, mainly directed towards correcting fixed deformity. To this end various types of tendon release are performed, including release of the thumb contracted into the palm.

Juvenile rheumatoid arthritis

Physiotherapy and hand splinting with drug therapy is the treatment of choice in childhood. Surgical joint reconstruction, synovectomy and tendon surgery may be considered in adolescence.

OCCUPATIONAL THERAPY FOR PATIENTS WITH CONGENITAL DEFORMITY

This is most appropriate in the area of detailed functional assessment, to help the surgeon decide on whether to operate and which operative procedure to adopt. Subsequently there may be a few weeks of remedial treatment, when splinting may be requested. The child must be encouraged to use both his hands, with provision of bilateral activities to achieve this. The parents must be made aware of the need to use both hands, otherwise the affected hand will not function to its full potential.

SPLINTING

In this small volume it is impossible to go into the subject of splinting in any depth, and some excellent books on the topic are listed at the end of this chapter.

As referrals will be received for splinting, the general principles will be covered. The work may be shared with an orthotist, a physiotherapist, or both.

It is essential that the referral is signed by the surgeon and gives specific instructions, as an unsuitable splint can cause real damage. The therapist must understand the underlying condition, the aims and implications of the splintage. Discussion between patient, doctor and therapist is also necessary after the splint is made.

The three types of splint are the resting (static) splint, the working (semi-dynamic) and the lively (dynamic) splint. The first two have no moving parts, but the lively splint uses hinges, elastic, rubber bands, spring wire and outriggers to move with the patient, assisting, correcting or resisting movement.

Resting splints are used to treat skeletal and joint problems. The purposes of resting splints are to:

- immobilize the joint(s) in the optimum position while healing takes place;
- support painful and inflamed joints and soft tissue;
- correct soft tissue imbalance, and prevent overstretching of weak tissues;
- prevent or correct deformity.

Working splints support the joints in their most functional position, and allow neighbouring joints to mobilize.

Lively splints are used in the treatment of kinetic problems, i.e. muscles, nerves, etc. They are supplied in order to:

- maintain joint mobility;
- replace lost function in damaged tissues and maintain tendon glide;
- prevent deformity by the prevention of adhesions and muscle contractures;
- correct deformity, including soft tissue imbalance and contractures;
- provide joint stability;
- restrict unwanted movement;
- remove accumulated oedematous fluid by the pumping action of muscles;
- maintain any improvement gained through therapy;
- strengthen movement through applied resistance.

Principles of splinting

The splint must maintain the optimum functional position, taking the anatomical arches of the hand into account. This position is with the wrist in 25° extension, the MCP joints in 40° flexion, the PIP joints in 30° flexion, the DIP joints in 10° flexion and the thumb in palmar abduction, but allowing the index finger to flex past it. The measurements are approximate guidelines.

If the hand is to be immobilized for a long time, it should be splinted in the 'safe position'. Ligaments should be on the stretch when the joints are immobilized, and to achieve this the MCP joints should be splinted in 90° flexion and the IP joints fully extended. The wrist is splinted in 30° extension, and the thumb in palmar abduction. This position is indicated for soft tissue injuries of the hand but is contra-indicated after nerve or tendon repair.

A working or lively splint must not extend beyond the palmar crease, as this will prevent normal movement of the MCP joints. Similarly, the bulk of the thenar eminence must be free and the edges of the splint flanged outwards so as not to impede thumb action. As much as possible of the palmar surface must be free, so as not to interfere with sensation.

The splint must not cause pressure over the areas where sensation is abnormal, nor over bony prominences. The dorsal aspect of the hand is vulnerable over the prominences of the MCP and IP joints, and the palmar surfaces of the MCP joints are vulnerable in rheumatoid arthritis. The metacarpal arch must be carefully supported, and any fixed deformity accommodated.

No joint should be needlessly immobilized. No part of the splint must impede circulation. If there are any incisions on the palmar surface, the digits should be placed in flexion and worked towards extension. If an incision is on the dorsal surface, splinting should be in the neutral position and the digits worked towards flexion and extension.

Mechanics of splinting

This applies particularly to dynamic splinting. Biomechanics is a science in itself and readers who wish to know more are referred to the work by Malick (1982). Basically, force produces movement in the form of compression, assistance or stretch, by the use of elastic materials or springs. The amount of pressure applied to correct deformity should be a little more than the pressure exerted by the deformity itself (Turner, 1981). Excessive pressure may cause ischaemia, nerve compression or skin ulceration. Pressure is reduced and friction eliminated by distributing the force over as wide an area as possible. Three points of pressure are required to provide balanced forces in splinting, e.g. the forearm-hand splint has a middle force supplied by the strap across the dorsum of the wrist, while the proximal and distal ends of the splint supply the counter forces. (Moran, 1986). The principles of leverage also apply, e.g. in the forearm-hand splint, the forearm trough supplies the force arm, the wrist forms the fulcrum, and the palmar pan acts as the resistance arm (Moran, 1986) (Figure 9.12).

Rigidity is important to avoid distortion. Curving the splinting material increases rigidity, e.g. the gutter of a forearm splint is half the circumference of the forearm. This should be two thirds the length of the forearm and flanged outwards at the edges to avoid pressure. A second layer of splinting material is often necessary to strengthen the wrist joint. A cylinder splint is the most rigid construction.

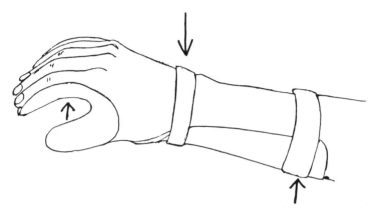

Figure 9.12 Palmar pan resting splint, showing three contact areas corresponding to the lever system of mechanics

Directional pull is important when splinting the fingers in flexion. Since the fingers converge in flexion, a finger flexion cuff (traction splint) should have each flexion assist individually adjusted to take account of the descent of the metacarpal heads towards the ulnar side, and the attachment should be close together on the palmar aspect at the wrist. If the fingers are pulled down straight, ulnar drift will occur on extension. Any finger hooks must be applied to the proximal half of the nail, to avoid levering the nails away from the nail beds.

Traction must be applied at 90° to the axis of the joint being mobilized, otherwise the finger cuff will cause pressure at one edge. High profile outriggers provide a better angle of pull than do low profile outriggers (Fess and Philips, 1987).

Design of the splint

Standard splint patterns should be used as a rough guide only, as each splint should be individually tailored to the patient. With regard to design, the patient's circumstances must be considered, e.g. if he lives alone he will have to put the splint on and off independently. If he works, it must be compatible with his job. It must be as simple and unobtrusive as possible, allow for optimum function, smooth fit, and do the job for which it was prescribed. The patient's skin condition and any altered sensation will affect the choice of material used.

Splinting materials

While the orthotist uses a variety of materials, the occupational therapist uses low temperature thermoplastics almost exclusively. The exception is plastazote, a high temperature thermoplastic for which a special oven is required. This makes a comfortable lightweight cylinder splint, but needs a reinforcing strip of vitrathene (another high temperature thermoplastic) for added strength. It is too bulky for any other hand splints, but is frequently used for cervical collars. It is very warm in wear.

Low temperature thermoplastics are softened in a hot water pan and moulded either over a thin stockinette tube or directly onto the skin. Different materials have different properties. Aquaplast and Orfit become transparent when they are ready for moulding, and the material sticks to itself readily and may stick to the pan. A few drops of detergent help prevent the latter. These materials are rigid when set. Orthoplast and Sansplint are less mouldable and may be easier for the inexperienced therapist to use. Orthoplast does not stretch or stick to itself. It is slightly pliable when set. Perforated thermoplastics allow for some cooling effect but a hole may coincide with a bony prominence and cause extra pressure, and in the stretchier materials the holes may enlarge too much and leave a weak spot.

Hexcelite resembles string vest material coated with thermoplastic. It is cool and lightweight but rather rough, so requires careful finishing and may be contra-indicated for patients with rheumatoid arthritis. It may have to be used in double thickness for strength, and it is springy.

Fitting the splint

Because the patient may be apprehensive, an explanation of the procedure re-assures him. If the patient is a young child, he may be allowed to mould a scrap of the splinting material himself to give him confidence. The patient should be seated comfortably, with his forearm resting on a clean towel on a table of suitable height. All tools and materials should be assembled in readiness and the splinting material manufacturer's instructions for use followed to obtain good results. After removal from the hot water, the splint is dabbed dry before application to the patient. The forearm section is wrapped around with crepe bandage from proximal to distal, and the thumb wrapped separately, to enable the therapist to concentrate on the hand section.

Use of gravity is helpful. A palmar splint can be applied and moulded with the forearm supinated, then before it sets, the arm and splint are turned over and the forearm trough moulded with the forearm pronated (Salter, 1987). If the forearm trough is moulded in supination, the forearm will migrate out of it in use (Moran, 1986). Gravity assists when fitting a dorsal splint in pronation.

The forearm must be correctly aligned with the third metacarpal, especially for an extension splint. The therapist then observes that the metacarpal heads form a line oblique to the axis of the forearm. Any clenching of the fist demonstrates the descent of the metacarpal heads towards the ulnar side. The splint should therefore be longer and higher on the radial side, and any outrigger bar should follow this oblique line and be positioned just proximal to the PIP joints.

The splinting material should be eased over bony prominences. Cutting a hole may increase pressure around the prominence and padding must be avoided as it alters the fit of the splint. Any crowding of the fingers in a palmar resting splint is remedied by the addition of interdigital ridges, which gives added strength through the girder principle.

In thumb splints, the web space must be maintained, with the thumb in wide abduction. If the aim is to increase the range of movement at the carpometacarpal joint, the force must be exerted on the metacarpal bone.

Finishing touches

After moulding, the splint should be re-applied to check for fit, tight areas eased using a heat gun, rough edges smoothed and all corners rounded. For comfort the splint may be lined with very thin self-adhesive material. Straps and reinforcements, etc. are attached according to the manufacturer's instructions. For hinges, one rivet is used; for straps, two rivets are needed. When using self-adhesive velcro, the thermoplastic is wiped with plaster solvent to take off the gloss, then the back of the velcro warmed with the heat gun before application to ensure stronger bonding. The use of velfoam or similar is convenient with velcro hooks, and the wider the strap, the less is the likelihood of undue pressure. Straps should be placed as near as possible to the ends of the splint, to hold it firmly in place and where they will not cause pressure. The best place for a wrist strap is just distal to the ulnar styloid. On completion, the splint should be fitted onto the patient and checked to ensure it achieves its objective.

Patient instruction

The patient must be warned to remove the splint if numbness or pins and needles occur, and to come back for adjustment of the splint. Any redness should subside within 20 minutes of removing the splint after wearing it for 30 minutes. If it does not, the splint needs adjustment.

Frequently the splint is worn in conjunction with an exercise programme, and should be easily removable for these sessions. The patient must be taught how to put the splint on and adjust it correctly, and he must be told when he is to wear it and when it is to be removed. He must be told that he may wash the splint in tepid water only, and not leave it in a hot place, e.g. a car window, otherwise it will distort. A written instruction sheet is helpful as a reminder.

The splint should be checked weekly to ensure correct fit. Unless the plan is very short term, periodic review is necessary, because changes in hand shape, etc. will alter the fit and the splint will need adjustment or replacement.

Splinting for specific conditions

For details on specific splinting, the reader is directed to the list of books at the end of the chapter.

COUNSELLING AND PSYCHOLOGICAL MANAGEMENT

Early in the chapter the versatility of the hand was discussed and attention drawn to the fact that the hand is very much on show. Impaired function, clumsiness and deformity are therefore much in evidence. The patient suffers from altered body image and both the functional disability and the outward appearance of the hand will cause emotional disturbance. People use both hands in most activities of daily living; there can be few jobs where the hands are not used to some extent, and socially the hands are very important. Therefore, the problem is forever making its presence felt. Many patients keep the affected hand in their pocket. It may not be used, resulting in an atrophied, stiff, possibly oedematous and non-functional hand.

If the patient injured his hand at work, he may have a compensation case pending which may delay recovery. The patient will be averse to returning to the place where the injury occurred. The patient with rheumatoid arthritis is probably concerned about the functional loss and developing deformity in his hands. The congenitally deformed patient usually has fewer psychological problems, as he does not suffer loss as such and has no alteration in body image. It is not until the child starts school that his problems arise, because of the natural cruelty of children to those who are 'different'.

The patient's family may also find it difficult to accept the effect on their member's hand, and may themselves need help. Counselling may therefore be desirable for both the patient and his family. The therapist may help the patient to consider and talk through his thoughts and feelings about his hand condition, releasing any pent-up feelings of resentment, anger or blame, and mourning the loss either of function or beauty of his hand. The main role of the therapist is to listen attentively and with empathy, allowing the patient to express his feelings, and not simply brushing them aside with a thoughtless 'cheer up' remark.

From the practical standpoint, the therapist can help the patient by teaching him to touch and explore the damaged area, or to study the deformity, thereby encouraging acceptance of it. The patient must be given the responsibility of caring for the hand. He may have to be helped in adjusting to a different role, lifestyle or employment. Most important, he must be enabled to be independent in daily living activities.

TOOLS FOR LIVING

Necessary tools will vary considerably, according to the cause of the hand condition. Tools which may be required for patients with rheumatoid disease are listed in Chapter 1. Children with congenital deformities readily adapt and rarely need gadgetry. The items most likely to be required are:

- tap turners;
- jar, bottle and can openers;
- adapted cutlery;
- Dycem matting;
- writing aids;
- flat tray purse;
- elastic shoelaces;
- handle adaptations, including angled handles, for implements at home and at work.

For information on:

1. *Hand Rehabilitation*   The books marked with an asterisk in the following lists.
2. *Splinting*   The books marked with a dagger in the following lists.

REFERENCES

Adams, J.C. and Hamblen, D.L. (1990) *Outline of Orthopaedics*, 11th edn, Churchill Livingstone, Edinburgh.

Bieber, E.J., Weiland, A.J. and Volenec-Dowling, S. (1986) Silicone rubber implant arthroplasty of the metacarpophalangeal joints for rheumatoid arthritis, *Journal of Bone and Joint Surgery*, **68-A**, no. 2, 206–9.

*Cailliet, R. (1986) *Hand Pain and Impairment*, 3rd edn, F.A. Davis, Philadelphia.

†Fess, E.E. and Philips, C.A. (1987) *Hand Splinting: Principles and methods*, 2nd edn, Mosby, St Louis.

Hofammann, D.Y., Ferlic, D.C. and Clayton, M.L. (1987) Arthroplasty of the basal joint of the thumb using a silicone prosthesis, *Journal of Bone and Joint Surgery*, **69-A**, no. 7, 993–7.

Hughes, S. (1989) *A New Short Textbook of Orthopaedics and Traumatology*, Edward Arnold, London.

Jensen, C.M., Boeck-Styns, M.E.H. and Kristiansen, B. (1986) Silastic arthroplasty in rheumatoid MCP joints, *Acta Orthop Scand*, **57**, 138–40.

†Malick, M.H. (1982) *Manual on Dynamic Hand Splinting with Thermoplastic Material*, 2nd edn, Hamarville Rehabilitation Center, Pittsburgh.

Moran, C.A. (ed.) (1986) *Hand Rehabilitation*, Churchill Livingstone, Edinburgh.

Moran, C.A. and Callahan, A.D. (1986) Sensibility, measurement and management, in C.A. Moran (ed.) *Hand Rehabilitation*, Churchill Livingstone, Edinburgh.

Peimer, C.A. (1989) *Arthroplasty of the Hand and Wrist: Complications and failures*, Instructional Course Lectures, American Academy of Orthopaedic Surgeons, Chicago.

Robins, R.H.C. (1986) Hand assessment charts, *Journal of Hand Surgery*, **11-B**, no. 2, 287–98.

*Salter, M.I. (1987) *Hand Injuries: A therapeutic approach*, Churchill Livingstone, Edinburgh.

Souter, W.A. (1987) Surgical management of rheumatoid arthritis, in S.P.F. Hughes, M.K. Benson and C. Colton (eds.) *Orthopaedics: The principles and practice of musculoskeletal surgery*, Churchill Livingstone, Edinburgh.

Swanson, A.B., Swanson, G. and Leonard, J. (1978) Post-operative rehabilitation programme in flexible implant arthroplasty of the digits, in J.M. Hunter, L.H. Schneider, E.J. Mackin and J.A. Bell (eds.) *Rehabilitation of the Hand*, Mosby, St Louis.

Turner, A. (ed.) (1981) *The Practice of Occupational Therapy*, Churchill Livingstone, Edinburgh.

*Wynn Parry, C.B. (1981) *Rehabilitation of the Hand*, 4th edn, Butterworths, London.

FURTHER READING

Alnot, J.Y. (1988) Wrist arthroplasties, in J.P. Razeman and G.R. Fisk (eds.) *The Wrist*, Churchill Livingstone, Edinburgh.

†Barr, N. and Swan, D. (1988) *The Hand: Principles and techniques of splintmaking,* 2nd edn, Butterworths, London.

Beckenbaugh, R.D. and Linscheid, R.L. (1988) Arthroplasty, in D.P. Green *et al.* (eds.) *Operative Hand Surgery, Vol.1*, 2nd edn, Churchill Livingstone, Edinburgh.

*Boscheinen-Morrin, J., Davey, U. and Conolly, W.B. (1985) *The Hand: Fundamentals of therapy*, Butterworths, London.

Browne, P.S.H. (1985) *Basic Facts in Orthopaedics*, 2nd edn, Blackwell Scientific Publications, Oxford.

Burt, A. (1986) Physiotherapy following joint replacements in the hand, *Physiotherapy*, **72**, 44–58.

Carter, P.R. (1991) *Reconstruction of the Child's Hand*, Lea and Febiger, Philadelphia.

Cooney III, W.P., Beckenbaugh, R.D. and Linscheid, R.L. (1983) Total wrist arthroplasty: problems with implant failures, *Clinical Orthopaedics and Related Research*, **187**, 121–8.

Dent, J.A., Smith, M. and Caspars, J. (1985) Assessment of hand function: a review of some tests in common use, *British Journal of Occupational Therapy*, December, 360–2.

Galley, P.M. and Forster, A.D. (1990) *Human Movement: An introductory text for physiotherapy students*, Churchill Livingstone, Edinburgh.

Laurence, M. (1980) Surgery, in G.S. Panayi (ed.) *Essential Rheumatology for Nurses and Therapists*, Baillière Tindall, London.

Leonard, J., Swanson, A.B. and Swanson, G. (1984) *Post-operative Care for Patients with Silastic Finger Joint Implants*, Orthopaedic Reconstructive Surgeons PC, Grand Rapids, Michigan.

McCombe, P.F. and Millroy, P.J. (1985) Swanson silastic wrist arthroplasty: a retrospective study of fifteen cases, *Journal of Hand Surgery*, **9-B**, No. 2, 199–201.

Meuli, H. (1983) Meuli total wrist arthroplasty, *Clinical Orthopaedics and Related Research*, **187**, 107–11.

*Mills, D. and Fraser, C. (1988) *Therapeutic Activities for the Upper Limb*, Winslow Press, Bicester.

Roberts, C. (1989) The Odstock hand assessment, *British Journal of Occupational Therapy*, July, 256–61.

Robinson, C. (1986) Brachial plexus lesions: management, *British Journal of Occupational Therapy*, May, 147–50.

Robinson, C. (1986). Brachial plexus lesions: functional splintage, *British Journal of Occupational Therapy*, October, 331–4.

Summers, B. and Hubbard, M.J.S. (1984) Wrist joint arthroplasty in rheumatoid arthritis: a comparison between the Meuli and Swanson prostheses, *Journal of Hand Surgery*, **9-B**, no. 2, 171–6.

Swanson. A.B. and Swanson, G. (1982) *Flexible Implant of the Radiocarpal Joint: Surgical technique and long-term results*, American Academy of Orthopaedic Surgeons Symposium on Total Joint Replacement of the Upper Extremity, Mosby, St Louis.

Trombly, C. (1983) *Occupational Therapy for Physical Dysfunction*, 2nd edn, Williams and Wilkins, Baltimore.

10

Bone tumours

A general practitioner meets on average only two cases of primary bone tumour in his career. It is, therefore, not surprising that frequently a bone tumour has become advanced before it is diagnosed, having been treated meanwhile as 'growing pains', osteo-arthritis or other more familiar conditions.

TYPES OF BONE TUMOUR

A tumour is a space-occupying lesion and is not necessarily malignant. Benign tumours, although symptomatic requiring removal, are not life-threatening and do not metastasize.

Osteoclastoma, more commonly called giant cell tumour (GCT), is usually benign but approximately 10% become malignant.

Primary bone tumours include chondrosarcoma, osteosarcoma, fibrosarcoma, Ewing's sarcoma, malignant GCT, and malignant tumours of bone marrow: myeloma and lymphoma.

PATHOLOGY

Chondrosarcoma is a tumour of cartilage, occurring mainly in the 30 to 60 year age group. It is found in the flat bones of the trunk and the ends of the long bones, more often the proximal ends. The patient complains of pain and swelling, sometimes occurring as a noticeable increase in size of a pre-existing lump. Radiographs show destruction of the cartilage with areas of calcification. This tumour grows slowly. It tends to metastasize late to the lungs. There is also a tendency to local recurrence. Radiotherapy and chemotherapy are not effective. Treatment is by radical excision or endoprosthetic replacement (EPR) of the diseased bone (*endo* = indwelling, *prosthetic* = artificial part).

Osteosarcoma is a highly malignant tumour, occurring in the 10 to 30 year age group, 50% of lesions appearing at the distal end of femur or proximal tibia. It affects the metaphysis, extending along the medullary cavity and eroding the cortex, eventually lifting or extending through the periosteum. The patient complains of constant non-mechanical pain, limps and presents with a hot, tender swelling. Radiographs reveal the typical picture of Codman's triangle

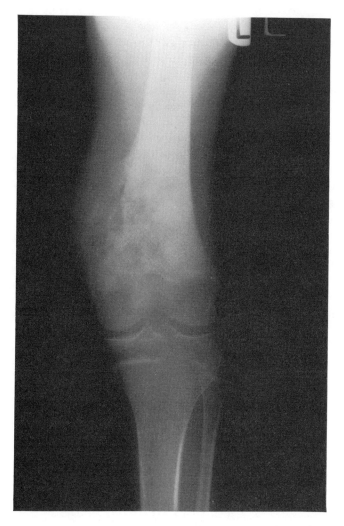

Figure 10.1 Osteosarcoma, showing sun-ray spicules on radiograph, as tumour penetrates periosteum, and Codman's triangle as the periosteum is elevated (reproduced by kind permission of the Bone Tumour Service, Royal Orthopaedic Hospital, Birmingham)

and sun-ray spicules (Figure 10.1). EPR may save the limb, or amputation may be necessary. Chemotherapy is prescribed but the survival rate is poor, only 50 – 60% of patients living beyond five years.

Parosteal sarcoma is a variation of osteosarcoma, arising from the periosteum, and does not usually extend into the medullary cavity. It is slow growing, and patient survival rate is 80% at five years. Treatment is by resection and occasionally chemotherapy. Paget's sarcoma is another variation of osteosarcoma occurring in about 1% of patients with Paget's disease, having a very poor prognosis, similar to radiation-induced sarcoma.

Malignant GCT is a tumour of young people between the ages of 20 to 40 years, usually not occurring until skeletal maturity. The majority of lesions are in the ends of long bones, especially the distal femur, proximal tibia and distal radius. The tumour extends up to the articular cartilage, rarely penetrating it. The lesion gradually expands the cortex without penetration. The patient presents with aching or discomfort and swelling. Treatment is by excision, sometimes with bone grafting, or by EPR. There is a tendency to local recurrence. Those GCTs which are malignant metastasize readily.

Ewing's sarcoma is a lesion within the bone marrow. It is very malignant, affecting children and young adults between the ages of 5 and 30 years. It spreads in the same way as osteosarcoma but is particularly permeative, extending along the medullary cavity of a long bone. It may also occur in the pelvis or ribs. The patient presents with pain, especially at night, with a hot, tender swelling, and may have general systemic symptoms such as fever and abnormal blood cell counts. Radiographs may show a typical 'onion skin' ossification as a result of periosteal elevation (Figure 10.2). Treatment is by chemotherapy,

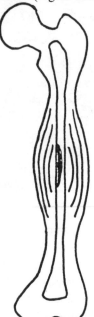

Figure 10.2 Ewing's sarcoma, showing 'onion skin' ossification

occasionally radiotherapy and surgery by major EPR or amputation. The survival rate is poor, only 50% living for a further five years.

Fibrosarcoma, now referred to as malignant fibrous histiocytoma, occurs in adults of all ages, but mainly in the 30 to 50 age group. It most often occurs towards the end of the shaft of the femur or tibia and may arise secondary to bone necrosis. The patient complains of pain, often followed by swelling or pathological fracture. Treatment is by chemotherapy and surgery.

Multiple myeloma is a malignant condition where there are a number of foci of bone destruction, most commonly in the vertebrae but also in the flat bones, upper ends of femur and humerus, and the skull. Radiographs show lytic or punched-out lesions, e.g. 'pepper pot skull'. The condition rarely occurs before the age of 40 years. The patient presents with pain, anaemia and general malaise. Treatment is by radiotherapy, chemotherapy and steroids, with spinal fusion or fixation of pathological fractures as appropriate.

Malignant lymphoma is a rapid-growing tumour of haemopoietic tissue, and affects all ages but the very young. It most commonly affects the pelvis and femur. If only bone is affected, the prognosis is better than when other lymphoid tissue is also involved.

Bony metastases are 40 times as common as primary bone tumours. They are bloodborne deposits of malignant cells, arising from a primary tumour in the breast, prostate, kidney or other organ. The patient may not have noticed any symptoms of the primary. The primary is sought out and treated first, but in 10–20% of cases the primary tumour is not found. The metastases commonly occur in the vertebrae, proximal bones, ribs and skull. Patients present with persistent pain and possible pathological fracture, which requires internal fixation. If the primary can be found and is treatable, treatment of a single bony metastasis may effect a cure. Otherwise the treatment for bony metastases is largely palliative, to prolong life and make it more comfortable. Chemotherapy is used, with radiotherapy for specific lesions.

Soft tissue lesions are included with bone tumours as the same team is best able to treat them, much being common to both conditions. Liposarcoma, a tumour of fatty tissue, and synovial sarcoma, a malignant condition of synovial tissue, are usually treated by wide excision.

'TUMOUR WORK-UP'

This is the protocol which the medical team follow when a patient with bone tumour is admitted to hospital, in preparation for the surgery which usually ensues. Urgent referral of bone tumours is desirable. It is important to diagnose the type and extent of the tumour quickly. In addition to taking a history of the case, diagnostic tests are commenced:

- radiographs of the affected area and the chest;
- blood tests, biochemical screen, liver function tests and serum proteins;
- bone scan to determine extent of the lesion and exclude other lesions in the skeleton;
- computerized axial tomography (CAT) or magnetic resonance imaging (MRI) scan to assess soft tissue involvement, and check lungs, etc. for metastases;
- biopsy for histological analysis.

From the results of these tests the medical team can determine whether surgery and/or chemotherapy may be beneficial. The oncologist and orthopaedic surgeon together make an individual plan of treatment, according to the patient's age, size, general physical condition and the type of tumour.

After biopsy, if the lesion is in the lower limb, the physiotherapist instructs the patient in the use of crutches, as the combined effect of the tumour and biopsy may have weakened the bone making a fracture possible if weight is borne on it. The patient continues non-weightbearing until surgery. Active exercise is contra-indicated, as tumours are vascular and increased blood supply to the tumour as a result of exercise could cause the tumour to metastasize, as well as increase the risk of fracture of a fragile bone.

If the tumour is of a type responsive to chemotherapy, treatment is commenced as soon as blood tests show the patient can withstand it. Three to five treatments, usually at three week intervals, are given prior to surgery. This may shrink the tumour, making it less vascular, making limb salvage surgery easier and safer. The size of the tumour is monitored and if it fails to respond, surgery may be performed earlier.

CHEMOTHERAPY

While patients treated by surgery alone have been found to have a 25% chance of survival to five years, those treated by combined surgery and chemotherapy have a 50% survival rate. The result with Ewing's sarcoma is even more encouraging; an increase in the survival rate up from 15% to 50%.

Pre-operatively, chemotherapy is used as above and is continued post-operatively to kill any occult micrometastases which may be present at the time of diagnosis. In the treatment of osteosarcoma, high dose methotrexate is used in conjunction with leucovorin, the first to inhibit multiplication of cells, the second to rescue normal cells. Vincristine may be used to promote the uptake of methotrexate by the cancer cells. Methotrexate crystalizes in acid urine, causing kidney damage, so sodium bicarbonate is given intravenously to alkalinize the urine. One of the alternative drug combinations is cisplatin and adriamycin. As many drugs cause nausea, anti-emetics are given initially.

Lorazepam given at the start of treatment enables the patient to sleep throughout, making it more tolerable.

These cytotoxic drugs have unpleasant and potentially dangerous side effects, the most noticeable being nausea, vomiting and hair loss. Bone marrow depression occurs and the patient's blood must be checked before each course to ensure that it has recovered from the previous course. Other side effects include allergy, diarrhoea or constipation, peripheral neuropathy, stomatitis, skin rashes, cardiac toxicity, pneumothorax and renal tubular necrosis. Prolonged treatment causes cirrhosis of the liver, other liver and renal disorders, defective osteogenesis and defective spermatogenesis. As a result of a low white blood cell count, resistance to infection is low and the patient must be protected from infectious diseases. Chickenpox and measles are very dangerous and should be avoided for six months after chemotherapy, although a prophylactic injection can be given if the patient is known to have been in contact with a person with these infections.

Strict precautions are taken in the preparation and administration of these drugs, to protect patients and staff, as they are very toxic.

RADIOTHERAPY

This may follow surgery for Ewing's sarcoma, myeloma, soft tissue sarcomas and some bony metastases. It may be used curatively or as palliation to ease symptoms.

SURGERY FOR BONE TUMOURS

This may involve scraping away the affected bone (curettage) or excising the affected area back into healthy tissue. If the tumour is aggressive or extensive, EPR of the diseased bone may enable the limb to be preserved. EPR is similar to joint arthroplasty with diseased bone being replaced by metal components, e.g. titanium or cobalt chrome alloy (Figures 10.3 and 10.4). The prosthesis is custom-made to the correct length and shape to fit the individual patient, ensuring that the limb is the same length as the contralateral limb. With the growing child, the parents' heights are used to estimate his ultimate height, and the prosthesis made in two parts which telescope together. It is lengthened at intervals by 6 mm at a time, by distracting the two ends and slipping a spacer between the two components.

The same surgeon should perform the biopsy and the definitive operation. The tumour is removed with an intact layer of healthy tissue with the biopsy scar, to eliminate contamination of the operative field. The prosthesis is inserted and fixed with bone cement. Soft tissues are sutured around the prosthesis, sometimes using a tube of terylene net. Reliance is then placed on a tube of scar tissue forming around the prosthesis for muscle attachment. This initial strength of muscle

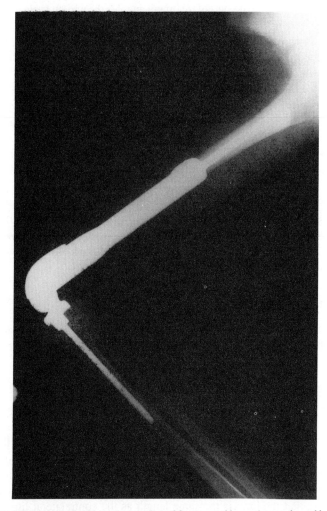

Figure 10.3 Endoprosthetic replacement of femur and knee (reproduced by kind permission of the Bone Tumour Service, Royal Orthopaedic Hospital, Birmingham)

attachment is therefore very fragile and must be treated with care. After closure of the wound no drains are used, nor interrupted sutures, to reduce the risk of infection which would prejudice the survival of the prosthesis.

Bone grafting may be employed to bulk up the bone following curettage or excision, with the ilium as the donor site. The fibula is frequently used for grafting and may be used to form strut grafts where considerable bone has been lost from the pelvis (Figure 10.5).

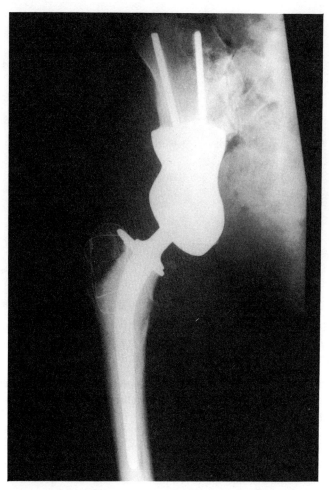

Figure 10.4 Endoprosthetic replacement of section of pelvis and hip joint (reproduced by kind permission ofthe Bone Tumour Service, Royal Orthopaedic Hospital, Birmingham)

The aim of surgery is to cure the patient. It may save the limb but if blood vessels, nerves or a neighbouring joint are involved in the tumour, the limb cannot be salvaged. Amputation is a last resort, either to save life or as a palliative measure to remove the source of severe pain. As advances are made in the treatment of bone tumours, amputations become fewer.

Results are encouraging. With osteosarcoma, if the patient survives the first two years, he stands an 80% chance of being alive five years later. The development of a good gait pattern depends on the patient's efforts and co-op-

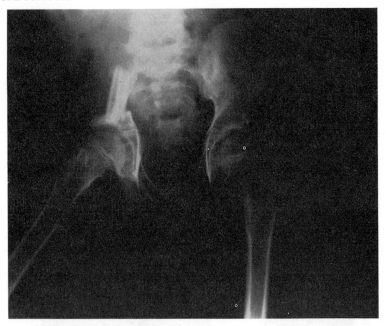

Figure 10.5 Fibular graft following excision of pelvic tumour (reproduced by kind permission of the Bone Tumour Service, Royal Orthopaedic Hospital, Birmingham)

eration with the physiotherapy programme. Loosening of the EPR after ten years may occur, but the EPR can be revised. Sometimes a knee prosthesis requires re-bushing, i.e. replacement of the polyethylene bush through the hinged prosthesis, through which the joint is bolted. As with joint arthroplasty, there is interest in uncemented prostheses which may decrease the chance of loosening.

Research continues into improved prostheses and techniques, use of allografts, better targetted drugs, radio-active isotopes which seek out metastases directly, etc. The increasing use of MRI scanning will enable earlier diagnosis and better surgical planning which in turn will improve the success of surgery, increasing the chance of survival.

THE CARE AND COUNSELLING OF THE PATIENT AND HIS FAMILY

If the reader considers the sections on tumour work-up and chemotherapy from the point of view of the patient and his family, it is clear that there will be great emotional shock. Contributory factors include:

- diagnosis of a dreaded disease;
- swift removal from familiar surroundings to hospital;
- diagnostic tests, some possibly frightening, certainly stressful;
- restricted activity, possibly bedrest, with resulting loss of dignity;
- chemotherapy, unpleasant and frightening, with up to four drip-stands round the bed;
- prospect of major surgery ahead;
- loss of earnings and other financial stress;
- anxiety about the effect of the illness on other family members.

Consequently every member of the treatment team must recognize the patient's distress, and be able to counsel him and his family. At the outset the medical team must explain the patient's treatment plan, allay unfounded fears and encourage his co-operation. Honesty is the best policy, so that the patient does not conjure up nightmares or unreal expectations. This lays the foundation for trust and prevents that trying situation when all concerned are avoiding the truth.

Staff must be prepared to take time over assessments and explanations. The patient will be anxious and want answers to many questions. He must be reassured that no question is too trivial to ask. The social worker may work especially closely with the occupational therapist at this point. The social worker's role is to offer practical help and support with socio-economic problems, and to encourage the patient and his family to express their distress, fear and anger. Any member of the rehabilitation team may be engaged in counselling, which involves non-judgemental listening to the patient and his family, and this in itself has a healing effect. The section on counselling in Chapter 1 is equally applicable to the tumour patient. He may need to go through the mourning process, because there may have to be some alteration to his lifestyle, e.g. a change of job or giving up a favourite sport. His body image will have altered, even if there is no marked alteration in his outward appearance. The temporary loss of hair alters his appearance, but a wig is supplied, although male patients tend to prefer wearing a cap.

PHYSIOTHERAPY

For each patient the physiotherapist makes an individual treatment plan, based on the muscles, etc. involved in surgery. She also carries out chest physiotherapy immediately after the operation.

After EPR of a bone in the lower limb, the patient exercises in bed. If the knee is affected, he is up after three days, but is on bedrest for two weeks if the proximal femur or pelvis is involved. Most patients are discharged about two weeks post-operatively, partially weightbearing, with a programme of exercises to follow at home. Six weeks after surgery the patient returns for one week of intensive physiotherapy, at the end of which he is fully weightbearing. Following curettage or bone grafting, he remains non-weightbearing for longer, to allow the bone to bulk up after curettage, or to unite after grafting.

If the shoulder or humerus is replaced, the elbow and wrist only are worked up to six weeks, then work commenced on the shoulder. If the rotator cuff is involved, the arm is immobilized across the chest initially and bandaged to the trunk if there is risk of subluxation. Mobilization proceeds more slowly and cautiously.

OCCUPATIONAL THERAPY

Occupational therapy intervention varies according to the surgery, the patient's circumstances and the prognosis. Patients with involvement of pelvis, proximal femur, spine, shoulder, elbow and forearm, especially of the dominant hand, may have daily living problems. When the lesion is from the knee downwards, occupational therapy intervention may be unnecessary, unless the bone has fractured and the patient is wearing a plaster cylinder.

Initially the occupational therapist should explain her specific role to the patient. On admission the patient may have no daily living difficulties but this may change following surgery. An elderly patient discharged on crutches to await surgery may be unable to negotiate stairs and be unable to reach her WC. In this case a bed downstairs and a commode may be called for. Even if there are no daily living problems at this stage, the patient is reassured that help is available should the need arise.

The occupational therapy assessment includes information concerning the patient's family support, his home facilities, and his employment and leisure interests. If surgery is imminent, it is wise to estimate what equipment will be necessary on discharge and alert the providing community agency so that they have the opportunity to assemble the items needed. Early discharge is normal and equipment must be provided immediately for the patient's security and protection.

Tools for living depend on the site of the lesion and the needs of the patient. If the hip joint is involved, provision should be made as for total hip replacement. If surgery involves the pubic ramis, the patient should be assessed for independence in rising from chair, bed and WC and bending to reach the feet. If pelvic reconstruction is to be performed, either by fibula strut graft or by EPR, the patient will be immobilized in a hip spica for six to 12 weeks. Necessary equipment may then include:

- single bed with monkey pole, downstairs;
- bedraising blocks;

- bedpan and waterproof mattress cover;
- commode if the patient can position over it;
- raised toilet seat, with dip side on patient's affected side;
- oval-to-round adaptor to position raised toilet seat as above on commode;
- Femicep urinal (for females);
- an extra-long reaching tool.

Toilet provision is a matter for individual assessment, as it depends on the patient's build and on the slight angle of abduction and/or flexion in which the hip is immobilized. Sitting is problematic, but a high-seated chair with a sloping back may suffice and the younger patient may manage to use a settee piled strategically with cushions, provided he has assistance with rising. The patient is mobile on crutches but unable to manage stairs. After the second stage of pelvic reconstruction when the EPR is inserted, no additional equipment is necessary.

When the upper limb is involved it is important to establish hand dominance. After surgery, the patient is more disabled for a time. The type of tools required may include a Manoy knife and plate, Dycem mat, bread buttering board, Belliclamp, etc. If he is using the clumsier non-dominant hand to manipulate them, the patient will need extra training in the use of these tools.

When spinal surgery is performed, provision of tools for living is as for spinal fusion. It must be made clear to the patient that any tools for living are intended as temporary aids and that he will be able to return all or most of them after his week of intensive physiotherapy. The older patient may need to rely on the raised toilet seat for longer.

Before discharge the patient's independence in dressing and grooming activities should be checked, and if he lives alone, he should practise making a hot drink and a snack. If family help is not forthcoming, he should be assessed for provision of home help and meals on wheels. After the intensive physiotherapy he should be able to prepare and cook a main meal, and should be assessed for safety and competence in doing this.

Time should be expended on the kitchen practice, the therapist sitting down and drinking a cup of tea or sharing a meal with the patient. This cosy, domestic situation encourages confidences in a relaxed atmosphere. The patient may reveal fears or previously unmentioned problems, so that steps can be taken to deal with them. Because of the severity of their pain before treatment, patients may have been aggressive towards family members and now feel guilty. Talking about it helps to relieve these guilt feelings.

The patient and his partner may come to the kitchen together, and once the drink has been made the therapist may withdraw, but be within calling distance. This enables the couple to talk, weep or console each other in the privacy which is lacking on the ward. The partner or family should be involved in the rehabilitation programme and the patient encouraged gradually to resume his former roles and interests. Contact sports are to be avoided, so another absorbing interest may have to be sought out.

Occupational therapy with the paediatric bone tumour patient

Much of the above applies equally to the treatment of children. The social worker supports the family network, since the parents are pre-occupied with the sick child. There may be other children at home who also need their parents' loving care. These healthy children may have guilt feelings or be jealous of the attention the sick child is receiving. The parents may feel guilty at giving less attention to their healthy children, and may be blaming themselves for the sick child's illness. Frequently the family's emotional suffering is as great as the patient's: theirs is the watching and waiting role, while the patient has the more active role to play in his own rehabilitation

Regarding daily living activities, teenage patients will have similar requirements to adults. They are inclined to shun much of the available equipment because of its connotations of abnormality, so only the most essential items may be accepted and these should be of a design which is as unobtrusive as possible. Few tools for living are required for younger children as they are very adaptable, have adults to wait on them and can more easily be lifted around. Many parents appreciate the provision of an outdoor wheelchair or buggy to enable them to cope; with other children at home, the mother is busy and the affected child cannot be left alone in the house while she shops and takes siblings to and from school.

Education is disrupted, as the child may have repeated episodes of hospitalization for chemotherapy and prosthetic lengthening surgery. Unless there is teaching provision within the hospital, it may fall to the occupational therapist to liaise with the younger child's teachers to provide schoolwork at the correct level, and to use play activities to facilitate normal psychosocial development and help the child express his fears and emotions. Education is an important issue for the adolescent, as it is difficult to provide the appropriate teaching in hospital at this level and future career prospects are at stake.

AMPUTATION

If there is a likelihood of amputation being necessary, the patient is warned before signing the consent form for surgery. Despite this, the reaction on recovery from the anaesthetic is one of shock and dismay and the rehabilitation team must encourage the patient to mourn for the limb in the same way as mourning the loss of a loved one. The patient feels a great sense of loss and worries as to how he will manage without the limb.

The sensitive attitude of the nurses and physiotherapists will help the patient through the early days. Their looking at and handling the stump without disgust and their confident attitude towards it help the patient's self-image. He must be encouraged to look at the stump, handle it and care for it early on, to enable him to accept the situation. Those who have never seen an amputation stump fear the sight, often imagining something grotesque. A good surgeon leaves an adequate flap of skin and muscle to close over the bone end, leaving it neat and well-padded to prevent soreness later.

Lower limb amputation

For eradication of a bone tumour, the below-knee site is the lowest likely to be encountered. Retention of the knee joint is a valuable asset, enabling easier fitting of a prosthesis and rendering it more functional. Disarticulation through the knee joint without severing the bone enables earlier fitting of a prosthesis. The mid-thigh or above-knee amputation produces an ideal stump for fitting a prosthesis. With each of these sites, the physiotherapist gives exercises to prevent the development of flexion contractures. If allowed to develop, such contractures prevent the patient weightbearing through the prosthesis. Lying prone helps to prevent this complication.

Disarticulation through the hip joint leaves no stump and the scar is anterior to the joint, so that the patient does not bear weight on it when sitting. Rehabilitation is easier than might be expected. Hindquarter amputation involves removal of the whole leg plus the ischium, pubis and all or most of the ilium. Again the scar is on the anterior aspect. Fitting of the prosthesis may be delayed for many weeks, depending on healing, the patient's physical state and any concurrent treatment.

Patients are mobilized quickly after surgery, standing out at about the second or third day, progressing to hopping with a walking frame after the high stumpless amputations, then onto crutches. Where there is a stump, a pneumatic post-amputation mobility (PPAM) aid is used within a week to maintain the walking pattern, and the massaging effect of this aid helps to reduce oedema. Physiotherapy aims to develop balance, maintain mobility in the remaining joints, prevent contractures, develop strong hip abductors and quadriceps muscles in below-knee amputations, strong hip abductors and extensors in above-knee amputation and improve power in the upper limbs.

The occupational therapist complements the physiotherapist's work, observing the patient's positioning and movement while assessing for independence, and reinforcing the physiotherapist's instructions.

The patient may prefer to sit on a soft seat, but sitting on a firm one prepares him for weightbearing on the ischium when he gets his prosthesis following hip disarticulation. As the ischial tuberosity is preserved after hip disarticulation, sitting is easier than after hindquarter amputation, when the patient's sitting balance is altered. A cushion made of calico filled loosely with polystyrene beads is helpful, the patient nestling into the cushion so that the spine is perpendicular. Checking the level of the shoulders is invalid: the spine may still be curved.

If the patient is in agreement, a wheelchair should be ordered early so that quality of life is improved by the ability to go further afield than is possible on crutches. Even after he has become proficient on his prosthesis, it is advisable for the patient to retain the wheelchair, as it may be needed if the prosthesis needs repair or if he develops stump problems. Because speed of provision is important at this stage in order to improve morale, a standard 8L wheelchair may be ordered with the rear wheels set back three inches for those with high amputation to balance the front of the wheelchair and prevent tipping due to the lost weight at the front. An 8BL is contra-indicated following high amputation since, even with the rear wheels set back, both the wheelbase and the castors are too small for this model to be sufficiently stable in use.

For the patient who is not to be fitted with a prosthesis, a more careful wheelchair assessment is necessary. The width should equal the width of the patient across the hips plus two inches, and the depth should measure the distance from the back of his bottom to the bend behind the knee minus two inches (5 cm). Lower backrests allow more arm function but offer less trunk stability. The seat height should be measured from beneath the lower thigh to the base of the shoe heel, plus an extra three inches (7.6 cm) for floor clearance. Use of a cushion affects the last measurement and affects the height of the armrests, which should be at the level of the forearms with the elbows flexed at 90°. Detachable armrests facilitate transfer, and desk-style armrests and a tray attachment are available. A model with larger castors is more stable.

The space available within the home must be taken into account when assessing for a wheelchair. Access needs to be ramped, with the maximum incline at 1 in 12. Doors must be at least 32 inches (81.5 cm) wide. Doors at right angles to narrow corridors may prove impossible to negotiate, the turning circle for a wheelchair being 60 inches (152.5 cm). It may help to rehang a door to open the opposite way, or on the opposite side of the frame, to obtain extra space. Bathrooms, being almost universally cramped, should have doors opening outwards.

Tools for living which may be needed after high level amputation depend on the patient's age, but may include:

- high seat chair, or raising device on existing chair;
- raised toilet seat and frame;
- bedraising blocks and possibly a monkey pole;
- commode and walking frame for night use;
- helping hand reacher;
- bath board, seat and non-slip mat.

The mattress must be firm, for ease of movement, for getting in and out of bed and to prevent flexion contractures. If the mattress sags, a fracture board must be placed beneath it.

Dressing problems as such are rare, but the patient should sit to dress as balance is affected. Kitchen practice is important because of altered mobility and the inherent hazards. The light workshop may be more appropriate for some patients to practise mobility while engaged in any activity other than pure walking. The patient should stand and walk as much as he can tolerate, using appropriate walking aids. When standing at a work surface there is a danger that, because the patient still feels the limb he will forget that it is no longer there, and may take a side-step onto the amputated side and fall. To prevent this, a stool should be provided at the correct height for the stump to rest on. It is useful if the patient can use the PPAM aid while he is in the occupational therapy department, so that his stance and gait may be observed to ensure that he maintains the correct patterns. He should stand erect and not develop the habit of leaning forward at the hips, and when walking should elevate the pelvis to swing the prosthesis through, avoiding swinging it out sideways. Figure 10.6 illustrates a flowchart for monitoring achievement of objectives following hip disarticulation or hindquarter amputation.

The patient is discharged home well before the prosthesis is supplied. The waiting time is variable, depending on healing, residual oedema, concurrent treatment, the age of the patient and his general fitness. It is helpful if the occupational therapist can give broad answers to the patient's questions concerning the future prosthesis. Except in the case of hip disarticulation or hindquarter amputation, a temporary prosthesis may be supplied initially to enable earlier weightbearing yet allowing for stump changes. The socket is the most important part of the prosthesis, as it is the part which comes into contact with the stump and through which the weight is borne. Total surface contact is the aim, to prevent congestion in the end of the stump. A woollen stump sock is worn to adjust fit and prevent chafing, a cotton sock to achieve finer fit and a nylon sock enables gliding to take place between stump and socket when the limb is being put on. Materials used in the making of prostheses are lightweight, hardwearing, rigid polypropylene, glassfibre laminate and flexible polymers, with a fairly natural appearance. They are body-powered in conjunction with gravity. Shoes with broad-based heels and non-slip soles are required and should be light in weight, as walking with a below-knee prosthesis uses 20% more energy and with an above-knee prosthesis 40% more energy than walking with two normal legs. With most prostheses it is necessary always to wear the same height heel, but the prosthetist can re-align the ankle to adjust the prosthesis and some models may be adjusted by the patient.

Training in the use of the prosthesis is carried out by a physiotherapist with specialist skills at the limb fitting centre. She teaches the patient to walk, manage stairs, transfers, etc. and how to get up from a fall.

OCCUPATIONAL THERAPY DEPARTMENT HIGH AMP.

NAME: NUMBER: DATE:

Pre-Op	Op.	Day 1	Day 2	Day 3	Day 4	Day 5	Day 6	Day 7	Day 8	Day 9	Day 10	Day 11	Day 12	Day 13 etc
Introduce self, check, home situation, accom, help, work, etc			As pre-op if not previously done											
Order wheel-chair													Check when wheelchair due for delivery ⟶	
						When pt. up to W.C. assess for adaptations			Monitor progress			Teach use of bath aids		
								When pt. sitting out provide cushioning		Monitor				Supply bead cushion if appropriate
									Preliminary referral to supplier of equipment					Detailed referral and expected discharge date ensure delivery of equipment
											Give NALD information			
												Kitchen assessment if appropriate	Probable home visit	
Monitor positioning and correct gait patterns while in OT's care														

Figure 10.6 Flow chart for use following hip disarticulation or hindquarter amputation

Upper limb amputation

This is much less common than lower limb amputation. The below-elbow and mid-humeral sites are more easily fitted with prostheses. The remaining joints of the affected arm must be mobilized to prevent development of stiffness or contractures. The physiotherapist puts the patient's two arms through the full range of movement at regular intervals.

If the amputation is through the shoulder joint (disarticulation), or a fore-quarter amputation in which the clavicle and scapula are removed along with the whole arm, disability is much greater. After disarticulation, the shoulder line is maintained and the prosthesis is useful. After forequarter amputation the shoulder line is lost, the new outline resembling a raglan sleeve. A simple lightweight prosthesis will be supplied to restore the shoulder line, and/or a cosmetic limb, useful only for positioning. Meanwhile it improves the patient's morale if the occupational therapist makes up a temporary shoulder pad of foam or plastazote. This may be encased in cotton fabric for comfort and is held in place inside a T-shirt with a dab of velcro. Similarly the patient who has undergone a scapulectomy will have a pronounced dropped shoulder line. For female patients, these operations cause problems with bra straps and fastenings. A sports bra with straps close together at the back may be suitable, otherwise the bra may be altered to a halter neckline and fastened at the front.

Independence in dressing is aided by the wearing of knitted fabrics, clothes with few fastenings or velcro tabs, elasticated waistbands, ties, laces, etc. Clothes management in the toilet may be aided by a woman holding up her skirt in her teeth, and a man using a button hook to fasten his trousers waistband. A cuddly thick bathrobe enables easy drying after a bath, and a suction nailbrush may also be used for brushing dentures.

Kitchen activities using a Manoy knife and plate, Dycem mat, bread buttering board, fixed potato peeler, Belliclamp, etc. encourage independence in cooking.

Following amputation of the dominant arm, fine skills must be built up in the remaining hand, because the prosthetic arm will be the assisting one. This is significant when planning return to work. The person with an academic or administrative job can manage reasonably well and the manual worker may cope adequately using his prosthesis. The person whose work requires precision, such as a draughtsman or a silversmith, may be seriously handicapped.

The patient is discharged home early and may become very proficient in the use of only one arm while he awaits his prosthesis. Well-motivated patients are ingenious in devising coping methods. Holding objects between the knees to position them, and use of the teeth, compensate to a large extent.

The patient will be asking questions about the prosthesis soon after the amputation, so it is helpful to know some answers. Cosmetic limbs are designed to improve the patient's body image and appearance, without attempting to improve function, e.g. those supplied following forequarter amputation. Body-powered prostheses use the remaining movement in the affected limb or, via a harness, use movements of the opposite limb. The greater the amount of limb removed, the less mechanically efficient is the prosthesis. There are specialized attachments for manipulating tools but the split hook is the most useful. A working prosthesis is also supplied with an interchangeable cosmetic hand. Electrically powered prostheses are becoming more popular and use rechargeable batteries. Since 1982, hybrid systems have been developed for above-elbow amputations. These are body-powered elbow mechanisms with myo-electric hand control, or servo-switch control attached to clothing. In myo-electric prostheses the electrodes are sited over the flexor and extensor muscles to obtain the required movement. It is usual for a body-powered prosthesis to be supplied first to accustom the patient to wearing one, and because it is lighter in weight. After an amputation, the patient is individually assessed and measured for his prosthesis, then re-assessed at intervals as the stump may alter in shape. The occupational therapist who treats the patient on the orthopaedic ward is unlikely to be the one who later trains him in the use of the prosthesis. Training in use of the limb involves activities of daily living, cookery, bilateral hand activities of all kinds, remedial and construction games, and heavier activities such as woodwork. In this way the patient learns to master use of the prosthesis in all kinds of situations, so that it becomes a part of him. Liaison with the school or workplace may also feature in the programme.

In the early days, if the amputation is at a high level, the patient learns to adjust to the altered balance. However the lost sensation on the affected side is a permanent disability, unlike the restoration of function which is achieved by provision of the prosthesis.

Stump pain

Pain in the stump end may be due to infection, adhesions, vascular problems or neuroma, and is solved with prompt medical attention. A neuroma is a mass of proliferated nerve fibres at the end of a severed nerve, and may be treated by local injection or occasionally by surgery. If stump pain persists, it may prevent the wearing of a prosthesis.

Phantom limb pain

This differs from stump pain in that it is felt beyond the amputation site. It is due to the sensory nerve endings in the stump producing an image of the amputated limb in the cerebral cortex. Its intensity varies and it may be permanent or transient. For most patients it gradually fades, but persists in some cases and may be severe. If the patient's pain was poorly controlled prior to amputation, the phantom limb pain tends to be related in intensity to the pain felt at that time. It may be helped by ultrasound, TENS, percussion over the stump, or by hypnosis. Once the prosthesis is fitted it becomes more acceptable, as the patient feels as if he is moving his own limb.

Altered body image

Where malignant disease is present, there are likely to be systemic symptoms such as weight loss, fatigue, pain and malaise. These may cause altered facial contours, body shape or physical function. Knowledge of the changes occurring within his body makes the patient anxious, depressed and apprehensive.

Surgery causes scarring: minor with a biopsy, major for a wide excision, mutilation following amputation. Chemotherapy causes hair loss and other side effects. Radiotherapy has local and systemic side effects, skin changes being common and very noticeable. This treatment is feared because of its associations with burns, radio-activity, sterility and radiation-induced cancers.

Even if the patient's body changes are not visible to the outside world, he knows of them. Body image, therefore, has two facets: the actual body changes, and the feelings the patient has towards them. The bodily alterations may be rapid, but the patient's adjustment to them is a much more gradual process.

Amputation is a devastating and disfiguring operation. Adjustment requires four distinct phases (Walters, 1981):

1. The impact of the knowledge that a limb must be amputated.
2. Retreat, during which the patient grieves for the loss of the limb.
3. Acknowledgement, as the patient becomes ready and able to take an active part in his rehabilitation.
4. Reconstruction, as the patient assumes responsibility for his own care and future development.

In order to help the patient progress satisfactorily through these stages of adjustment, five steps have been suggested (Donavon and Pierce, 1976). The patient should be encouraged to:

1. accept the appearance of the operation scar;
2. touch and explore the area;
3. learn to care for the scar;
4. become independent in daily living activities;
5. accept his altered appearance, if necessary adjusting his lifestyle.

The patient should be prepared for the ordeal of facing the outside world again, because within the hospital he is in a sheltered environment. It may help him to discuss how he will explain his amputation to others. The next step may be venturing out of the ward to the hospital shop, then perhaps an outing to a local café or pub, accompanied by a supportive relative or therapist. The longer he holds back from meeting the world at large, the harder is the adjustment.

Amputation is especially devastating to the adolescent. Physical appearance is tremendously important to him, and he is already struggling with emotional and physical changes. As a result of the surgery and possible chemotherapy, he has to depend on his parents longer than he would wish, and frequent periods of hospitalization interfere with his educational and social development. Previous plans for a career and involvement in sports may have to be modified or abandoned. The whole family needs support and the therapeutic team must encourage a positive attitude towards rehabilitation and supply accurate information. The most acceptable fragment of information for an adolescent bone tumour patient in receipt of Mobility Allowance is that he is legally entitled to drive at the age of 16.

Sexual counselling

If a person looks good, he tends to feel good, and vice versa. This is important regarding sexual attraction, therefore the adolescent who has had an amputation must make a special effort over his dressing and grooming. This will improve his self-image and confidence, and largely overcome the initial disadvantage.

If the patient already has a partner, both are likely to be frightened of the effect of scarring or mutilation. To one who is scarred, touch by a loved one is important for his security and self-esteem. Some people are repelled by scars and stumps and need help in overcoming this.

Couples may experience great difficulty in resuming relationships. Fatigue or pain may reduce the sex drive. Anxiety or the effects of treatment can cause impotence or frigidity. If the patient requests any information concerning sex, staff should either supply the information, or point the patient towards a source of help. A marriage guidance counsellor or SPOD are valuable contacts. To enable embarrassed people to seek help, the addresses of these two organizations should be displayed in a patients' circulation area.

Chemotherapy and radiotherapy have a damaging effect on fertility, and prior to treatment young men are offered the facility of a sperm bank so that they may still father a child.

SUPPORT GROUPS

The social worker may obtain funding for equipment, holidays, travel to and from hospital, etc. on the patient's behalf, from the Malcolm Sargent Cancer Fund for Children up to the age of 18 years, and for adults from the Macmillan Fund.

The BACUP and Cancerlink organizations provide information and support for patients and their carers (addresses in appendix). The National Association for Limbless Disabled produce a magazine for members and provide a network of people who have themselves experienced amputation, who will empathize with and encourage new amputees.

THE ROLE OF THE OCCUPATIONAL THERAPIST WITH THE TERMINALLY ILL PATIENT

On occasion the prognosis is very bleak, and the patient is diagnosed as terminally ill. He may or may not remain on the orthopaedic ward, but the occupational therapist will at least initiate a programme for his benefit. This is somewhat of a volte-face for the therapist, as her goal is usually improvement and/or independence for the patient. It is possible for the rehabilitation team to overlook the patient who is not going to recover, leaving him feeling abandoned. Occupational therapists, having studied the physical and psychological aspects of human occupation, are uniquely able to contribute to the care of the terminally ill. Attainable goals may be set, leading to improved quality of what remains of life.

The patient and his family have first to come to terms with the prognosis. Unless they are aware of the terminal nature of the illness, it is impossible to follow a realistic programme. Elizabeth Kubler-Ross (1969) described the stages through which an individual passes on learning tragic news: denial and isolation, anger, bargaining with fate, depression and finally acceptance. Both patient and family members are involved in this process.

Often the victim of a bone tumour is young and has just realized how much life has to offer. It is then especially hard to come to terms with the prognosis, particularly if the patient does not yet feel ill. Denial of anxiety is abnormal and staff must be aware that deep down the patient is anxious. Feelings of anxiety may be suppressed by excessive talking, either to prevent his mind dwelling on his fate or to prevent others talking about it. Early on anger may be displayed, but as physical energy wanes, depression replaces anger. If the patient can be encouraged to complete outstanding tasks, he is more likely to settle into a mood of acceptance. Referral to occupational therapy is a positive step, encouraging hope which is essential to survival, but false hopes must not be raised.

The patient can become childish and demanding to cover up the unacceptable and degrading process of physical deterioration. He fears becoming a burden on his family. Loss of familiar roles is painful and the whole family have to adjust to their changing role relationships. If the patient loses his social role, he may become isolated to the point of feeling worthless. Occupational therapy intervention evaluates what prevents the patient carrying out his previous activities, and will take into account:

- the patient's role within the family;
- the patient's socio-economic role;
- functional problems, maximizing areas where function is unimpaired;
- effects of treatment and fatigue;
- what has been most important to the patient in his life, and what he would still like to achieve.

A plan of action is now possible. The patient's involvement in making this plan is vital. It gives him a feeling of control, lacking in his previous treatment. Family members should be incorporated into this programme, to help them adjust to the altering circumstances. They must be reassured that their fears, frustrations and even resentment are normal. Open communication is important and the therapist herself may express feelings of sadness, to empathize with the group. Her own approach should be quietly positive and moderately cheerful, but not overly so, as this displays a lack of sensitivity and professional confidence.

The goals of oncology rehabilitation have been divided into four parts (Dietz, 1981):

- prevention of potential disability;
- restoration to pre-morbid levels of activity;
- support through the stages of progressive disease;
- palliative treatment to prevent complications during increasing disability.

The last two goals may be summed up as enabling the patient to live to the full what remains of his life. Key tasks include maintenance of independence by whatever tools are necessary. Quickly provided housing adaptations such as handrails and halfsteps may be of benefit. Chair and bedraising blocks may maintain independence and dignity. Prevention of a housebound existence by means of a wheelchair, plus portable ramps, may enable the patient to come and go independently. All of this gives the patient some control over his environment and reduces his feelings of being a burden on his family. Advice on energy conservation (Chapter 1) will help to alleviate the fatigue inherent in terminal illness. Relaxation methods (Chapter 11) may help to relieve pain and stress.

The use of activity maintains strength, co-ordination and dexterity, and engages the patient in a meaningful task, promoting self-esteem and mastery of his environment. This meaningful task must relate to the patient's satisfying achievements in the past, and fulfil some ambition for his remaining lifespan. The carer should have a contingency plan for coping with the patient if he attempts too much. If it is his work which gives the patient the greatest satisfaction, the aim should be to keep him there as long as practicable.

Pain is controlled by opiates, given before the pain returns. In this way a lower dose is needed, side effects are avoided and addiction does not occur.

Once the correct dose is found, pain is controlled and the mind remains clear. If the pain increases, the dosage is increased accordingly.

Care and support of staff dealing with the terminally ill

Staff who work with the terminally ill are prone to stress. It is inevitable that staff are saddened by the decline and death of patients they have come to know well. If staff become irritable, find it hard to concentrate, begin to smoke or drink more heavily, sleep badly, have digestive disturbances or find it hard to 'unwind', they are suffering the effects of stress. It is important to recognize this and to take time to withdraw and talk it over with people who understand, usually fellow workers. If staff do not acknowledge their own grief they become unable to cope with the demands made upon them. Their personal and domestic life may also suffer. This can lead to a breakdown in the situation, when they have to leave the job.

Apart from the mutual support among the team members, a formal support network may be desirable, under the auspices of a trained counsellor. Above all, it is essential that each team member has an absorbing outside interest that refreshes and restores them. This enables staff to become more closely involved with and supportive towards the patients while they are present with them, without detriment to their own physical and mental health.

REFERENCES

Dietz, J.H. (1981) *Rehabilitation Oncology*, Wiley, New York.
Donavon, M. and Pierce, S. (1976) *Cancer Care Nursing*, Prentice Hall, London.
Kubler-Ross, E. (1969) *On Death and Dying*, Macmillan, London.
Walters, J. (1981) Coping with a leg amputation, *American Journal of Nursing*, **81**, 1349–52.

FURTHER READING

Boren, H.A. (1985) Adolescent adjustment to amputation necessitated by bone cancers, *Orthopaedic Nursing*, **4**, no. 5, 30–32.
Brown, P.S.H. (1985) *Basic Facts in Orthopaedics*, 2nd edn, Blackwell Scientific Publications, Oxford.
Davies, M. (1988) Sexual problems and physical disability, in C.J. Goodwill, C. John, and M.A. Chamberlain (eds.) *Rehabilitation of the Physically Disabled Adult*, Croom Helm/Sheridan Medical, London.
Downie, P.A. and Kennedy, P. (1981) *Lifting, Handling and Helping Patients*, Faber, London.

Ham, R. and Cotton, L. (1991) *Limb Amputation*, Chapman and Hall, London.

Hambrey, R.A. and Withinshaw, G.(1990) Electrically powered upper limb prostheses: their development and application, *British Journal of Occupational Therapy*, January, 7–11.

Hughes, S. (1989) *A New Short Textbook of Orthopaedics and Traumatology*, Edward Arnold, London.

Humm, W. (1977) *Rehabilitation of the Lower Limb Amputee*, 3rd edn, Baillière Tindall, London.

Lloyd, C. (1989) Maximising occupational role performance with the terminally ill patient, *British Journal of Occupational Therapy*, June, 227–9.

Luff, R. (1988) Amputations, in C.J. Goodwill and M.A Chamberlain (eds.) *Rehabilitation of the Physically Disabled Adult*, Croom Helm/Sheridan Medical, London.

Melzack, R. *et al.* (1988) *Challenge of Pain*, rev. edn, Penguin Books, Harmondsworth.

Nichols, P.J.R. *et al.* (1980) Rehabilitation following amputation, in *Rehabilitation Medicine: The management of physical disability*, 2nd edn, Butterworths, London.

Oelrich, M. (1974) The patient with a fatal illness, *American Journal of Occupational Therapy*, **28**, no. 7, 429–32.

Price, B. (1986) Keeping up appearances, *Nursing Times*, **82**, 58–61.

Salter, M. (1988) *Altered Body Image*, Wiley, Chichester.

Stedeford, A. (1984) *Facing Death*, Heinemann Medical Books, London.

Strong, J. (1987). Occupational therapy and cancer rehabilitation, *British Journal of Occupational Therapy*, January, 4–6.

Tigges, K.N., Sherman, L.M. and Sherwin, F.S. (1984) Perspectives on the pain of the hospice patient: the roles of the occupational therapist and physician, in P. Cromwell (ed.) *Occupational Therapy and the Patient with Pain*, Haworth Press, New York.

11

Pain control

Pain may be classified into three types: intermittent, acute and chronic. The orthopaedic patient is prone to all three types to some degree, and while the orthopaedic surgeon can abolish or relieve pain in many situations, a significant number of patients have to learn to live with their pain. Such is the nature of the pain of rheumatoid arthritis, metastatic bone disease, phantom pain following amputation and some back pain. There also arises the situation where a patient admitted for joint replacement is found to be medically unfit for surgery, and is discharged still in pain. With these cases there is clear physiological reason for the pain.

Acute pain has its uses. It tells us when something is wrong, so that we can protect ourselves from danger or take remedial action. Magdi Hanna (1988) lists five characteristics of acute pain:

- The cause is known and recognizable.
- The pain is of no more than a month's duration.
- Pain is accompanied by anxiety.
- Treatment is fairly simple and effective.
- The outcome is complete cure.

Magdi Hanna lists the following characteristics which distinguish chronic benign pain:

- The cause is difficult to diagnose.
- Pain is of long duration, possibly for years.
- The patient is depressed, with probable behaviour and personality changes.
- Treatment is complicated and may require a combination of methods.
- Complete cure is rare.

Pain is a subjective experience and different people have differing levels of pain tolerance. This may be influenced by childhood attitudes towards pain, cultural background and personality type. This last is the indecisive, diffident person, who may enjoy receiving sympathy and concern and uses pain as an excuse to escape from difficult situations.

Chronic pain persists after the original condition has cleared and the warning signs are no longer useful. The body's response to pain is similar to the stress response. If this state of affairs becomes chronic it becomes an illness in itself. The patient develops pain behaviour: groaning, grimacing, poor posture, attention seeking and inactivity. The pain wears him down, he is depressed, debilitated, neglects his appearance, does not eat or sleep well, moves little, takes no interest in his surroundings, and his relationships with family and colleagues are adversely affected. His status becomes that of an invalid. Brena (1978) lists five sequelae seen in chronic back pain, regardless of its presumed cause: drug dependency (takes 'pills although they do no good'); decreased function; disuse (loss of power and flexibility); depression; and disability (inability to work or carry out normal daily living activities). Cailliet (1988) describes this cycle as SAD, i.e. Somatic, leading to Anxiety, leading to Dependency and disability.

This chronic pain syndrome does not improve, nor does it tend to progress. As there is no apparent physical cause for the pain, the surgeon is inclined to abandon the patient or refer him to a psychiatrist, both of which are likely to cause resentment.

If compensation for a back injury is pending, the doctor may suspect the patient's motives, so the patient may exaggerate the symptoms to try to convince the doctor of his pain. This makes diagnosis difficult and may lead to distrust between doctor and patient. Jayson (1987) writes that there is no evidence to support the view that 'compensation neurosis' is a common occurrence.

The patient with chronic pain syndrome may be admitted onto the orthopaedic ward for assessment. He must be treated with patience and understanding. It is important to gain his trust and co-operation, and counselling skills are essential. In addition to the above characteristics, the patient talks interminably about his pain, and as each possible solution fails, he grows more despondent.

Although a complete cure is rare, some forms of treatment can relieve the problem. Melzack and Wall (1988) list four major approaches to the relief of chronic pain: pharmacological, surgical, sensory and psychological. While she will be actively involved in the last of these, the occupational therapist will find a background knowledge of the other three useful.

THE PHARMACOLOGICAL APPROACH

This includes the administration of analgesics and NSAIDs. If pain is continuous, analgesics are given at regular intervals before the pain returns. If the pain is worse at certain times, the analgesic is given 20 minutes before the pain is due. Indomethacin suppositories bypass the stomach and are more slowly absorbed, so give longer term pain relief. These drugs act directly on inflamed tissues.

Narcotic drugs act by interfering with the transmission of pain signals between the brain and the painful area, and include opium and morphine. Morphine acts in a similar way to the endorphins released by the mid-brain, inhibiting pain. A placebo may be beneficial, as it may cause the release of endorphins. According to Melzack and Wall (1988), a survey showed that 75% of patients experienced pain relief from morphine, while 35% of patients given placebos experienced pain relief, large placebos being more effective than small and two placebos being more effective than one!

Tranquillizers may be used in conjunction with mild analgesics to reduce anxiety and promote relaxation. Anti-depressants may be used to relieve anxiety and to act as a night sedative.

THE SURGICAL APPROACH

Nerve block injection, using guanethidine, block the action of noradrenaline secreted at the sympathetic nerve endings, thus relieving pain, while the sensory fibres are not affected. Sympathectomy is another method, where a long needle is used to reach the sympathetic nerve ganglia. A local anaesthetic is used first to test that the right area has been located, then a destructive fluid such as alcohol is injected.

Neuro-stimulators may be implanted for the relief of intractable pain, especially where a nerve had been irreparably damaged. Minute electrodes are implanted in the epidural space, usually in the thoracic spine. Wires running just beneath the skin are connected to a tiny generator, which is powered by long-life batteries. The system works by closing the 'pain gate', and it also increases the blood supply to the area. In a very small minority of cases a neuro-stimulator is implanted in the brain, where it appears to encourage endorphins, but since the procedure carries a high risk it is rarely performed.

THE SENSORY APPROACH

This is the approach of the physiotherapist and includes massage, manipulation, traction, use of superficial heat, ice packs, and TENS. This last uses the 'gate control' theory of pain. It is thought that neural mechanisms in the dorsal horns of the spinal cord control the flow of nerve impulses from the periphery to the cord cells that project to the brain, acting like a gate. Part of the theory is that larger, faster conducting fibres carrying sensation can block the impulses from the smaller, slower conducting fibres carrying pain, so that the modulatory influence of the 'gate' affects the somatic input before the pain is perceived. The process is similar to the jamming of a radio signal. The TENS equipment consists of a small box with batteries and controls to regulate the power and frequency of impulses. Electrodes attached to the site causing the pain aim to close the 'pain gate' via sensory nerve pathways. Over 50% of patients obtain long term relief of pain with this treatment. TENS machines interfere with the function of cardiac pacemakers and may also affect heart rhythm in some patients, hence the warning signs in physiotherapy departments.

The sensory approach also includes acupuncture, which relieves symptoms but does not treat the cause of the pain. It may help by closing the 'pain gate' or by causing the release of endorphins in the brain.

THE PSYCHOLOGICAL APPROACH

Because of the physical and psychiatric input in her training, the occupational therapist can play a large part in the rehabilitation of the chronic pain sufferer. It does require time and patience in listening attentively to the patient at the outset. Counselling plays an important part, listening to the patient's outpourings, which will probably release a great deal of anger and resentment. There is little need to talk back to the patient, other than to make a comment to show that he is being understood or to ask whether you have understood correctly by repeating what has been said. Observation of his body language is important to gain additional information, which may be used in the treatment plan. Examples of this are tension and grimacing, indicating pain. Movement patterns, e.g. walking, getting in and out of a chair, reaching for objects, etc., also give a clue as to pain level.

THE OCCUPATIONAL THERAPIST'S ROLE

The occupational therapist assesses the patient's home situation, obtaining details of any family living at home and what support is available. This may reveal whether there are problems within the family. If the patient works, information is gleaned as to what activities are involved, what job satisfaction is gained, and whether the patient is resentful or angry if he feels that the work was the original cause of his illness. The psychological damage caused by injury is often as disabling as the physical damage. It is also helpful to know if the patient was a hypochondriac prior to the onset of pain. Discussion concerning the family and work roles will demonstrate how the patient's self-image is affected, and enquiry into his leisure interests will indicate how his social role has altered.

Having elicited this information, goals should be set. These include the re-establishment of occupational roles within the family and employment, and resumption of leisure interests. Increasing achievement in these areas leads to increased confidence and self-esteem. The means of achieving these goals include:

- assessment and instruction regarding difficult activities of daily living;
- education in proper body mechanics;
- increasing activity levels;
- counselling;

- relaxation training and stress management;
- work assessment and resettlement.

Each of these treatment areas may be applied to any form of chronic pain, but the problems in daily living activities are possibly more relevant to chronic back pain than to any other condition, and the section on tools for living in Chapter 5 suggests solutions. However, it must be remembered that the patient's pain has passed its useful purpose, so the fuller details on coping with acute back pain should not be communicated, otherwise the chronic pain syndrome may be reinforced.

Education in proper body mechanics has been covered in Chapters 1 and 5, regarding rheumatoid arthritis and back pain respectively.

Increasing activity levels should be a gradual process, related to the patient's interests and occupational roles. The principles of proper body mechanics should be employed when carrying out activities. The length of time spent in activity and the required energy output should both be increased. Treatment may be on an individual or group basis. The latter is useful in improving socialization and discouraging pain behaviour.

While assessing and treating the patient, the opportunity for counselling may arise spontaneously and the opportunity should be grasped. The family may need to be involved if their co-operation is needed for more effective treatment.

Work assessment and resettlement are discussed in Chapter 12.

Relaxation training, especially in group sessions, is a valuable therapy. Stress management is closely related but also involves observation of what increases pain, and at what time of day pain is at its worst. Active periods may then be timed when the pain is more tolerable, and triggering situations avoided as far as possible.

Relaxation helps to control pain in several ways. It gives the patient something positive to do and the activity distracts the mind from pain. Also, pain causes tension and muscle guarding to protect the area from further pain. If relaxation can be induced, muscular tension is reduced, blood flow is increased and relief from pain ensues.

Relaxation techniques

By lying down to rest, weight and pressure are taken off the intervertebral joints and discs, allowing healing. If a suitable position is adopted, tense muscles relax and pain is relieved. Patients will find different positions suit their individual needs, but the following may be tried:

- Lie on the back on a firm base, with no more than one pillow.
- As above, but support the lumbar curve by placing a small pillow or folded towel in the hollow.

- Lie with several cushions under the calves, with hips and knees at right angles, or the same position with the calves resting on a cushioned chair seat. This flattens the lumbar lordosis and is termed the Fowler's position.
- Side-lying, with a pillow between the legs to prevent the spine twisting. A second pillow may be needed in the waist hollow.

If the patient finds a sitting position which is relaxing, this is acceptable. The spine and limbs must be well supported.

Having achieved a comfortable position, the patient can be instructed in any of the following relaxation techniques:

1. The alternate muscle tighten, muscle relax method, starting with the feet and working upwards, ending with the facial muscles. The patient finally rests in a relaxed state, breathing slowly and easily, using the abdominal muscles for breathing in preference to the chest muscles. Breathing out through the mouth and with the lower jaw relaxed greatly aids relaxation throughout.
2. The patient closes his eyes and concentrates on his breathing. He then focuses on the thought 'My left arm is heavy' for a time, then repeats this procedure with each limb in turn. If he repeats the procedure with 'My left arm is warm,' etc., the process can lead to an increased flow of blood to the area, with beneficial effect. This is a kind of self-hypnosis and may be carried through to concentration on a thought such as 'My pain has almost gone.'
3. The playing of soothing music may help a patient to relax. This is a very personal choice, so great care must be taken if working with a group, otherwise increased tension could be the end result!

A simple myographic biofeedback machine attached to the fingertips may help the patient to learn to control his tension at will. The machine works by measuring electrical skin resistance. With the electrodes on the fingertips, the machine emits a loud sound when the patient is tense and goes quieter the more relaxed he becomes. He learns how to reduce his tension by whatever means suits him best. If he is told at the outset that the machine will help to relieve his pain, it has a placebo effect.

Coping strategies

Melzack and Wall (1988) list six coping strategies for dealing with chronic pain:

- Imagine you are somewhere pleasant.
- Imagine the pain is trivial, e.g. tingling rather than pain.
- Imagine the pain is due to a different, exciting cause.

- Concentrate on external matters instead, such as a specific task or watching a specific event.
- Focus the attention on reciting a poem or doing some mental arithmetic.
- Focus on the pain, but as if you are about to write an article on it, so that you are detached from the pain itself.

Particular procedures suit different kinds of pain and different personalities. These coping strategies may make the pain more bearable, but do not abolish it. Two or more methods combined are more effective. The second strategy has proved most helpful in coping with severe pain, e.g. the pain of amputation or rheumatoid arthritis.

Guided imagery

This technique, described by Broome and Jellicoe (1987), is an elaboration of Melzack and Wall's first coping strategy. The patient can learn to divert his attention from pain by picturing himself elsewhere, such as by the sea on a summer day, or in a quiet wood, or beside a log fire in a cosy room. By this means he takes himself out of the pain situation and into a new painfree place.

Meditation

This is a different type of meditation from religious contemplation. There are several methods, and again different methods suit different personalities. The occupational therapist's objective is to get the patient to relax, and the aim of meditation is to concentrate on a distracting object, sound or word to the exclusion of all other thoughts.

Traditionally the lotus position is adopted for meditation, but the patient with chronic pain must adopt a position which is comfortable for him. In a quiet place he focuses his attention on one of the following:

- an imagined object, e.g. a star, diamond, etc.;
- a real object directly ahead of him, e.g. a candle flame;
- a sound rhythmically repeated, e.g. 'omm, omm';
- a colour, or colour range, perhaps passing through the colours of the spectrum.

Initially concentration may be maintained for only a very short time before other thoughts intrude. With practice, the time will be gradually extended and will induce relaxation, and in some cases can cure psychosomatic illness (Chaitow, 1985).

Tactile meditation is another technique. A set of worry beads or a few smooth rounded pebbles are used for this, and are held loosely in one hand while the other is used to move them slowly and rhythmically through the fingers, consciously feeling each one, counting them and listening to the sound they make. This should be pursued for about ten minutes.

A similar method is based on an old Oriental proverb, 'Whatever you are doing, enjoy doing it'. The occupational therapist can guide the patient through a simple task, e.g. peeling an apple, washing the hands, picking a rose, etc. For example, select the finest rose, cut the stem carefully, study the thorns and ponder on their purpose, note the glossy leaves, revel in the colour, shape and scent of the flower and stroke its velvety petals. All other thoughts should be excluded while doing this, the patient completely absorbed in the task, reducing stress, distracting the mind from pain and gaining more satisfaction from life.

Broome and Jellicoe, two clinical psychologists, have written a self-help guide to pain management (1987). It is directed at people who are motivated to help themselves, and includes asking themselves searching questions such as, 'Is this loss of interest only because of the pain, or are there other causes?' and 'Do I sometimes use the pain as an excuse not to do something I dislike doing?'. It helps patients to understand and monitor their pain, explains relaxation techniques and goal setting, and may be recommended to patients to back up the treatment they are receiving.

Any of the foregoing techniques may be taught by the occupational therapist, and once the patient has discovered which method best suits him, he can continue with his own treatment, giving him a sense of mastery over his illness.

ALTERNATIVE MEDICINE

Acupuncture has already been mentioned in the section on the sensory approach. Hypnosis can be of value in this context, although relatively few people can be helped. Only 30% are deeply susceptible to hypnosis, with another 30% being moderately susceptible (Melzack and Wall, 1988). Relaxation precedes hypnosis and the process lowers the blood pressure and slows the metabolic rate. Given the patient's trust, the hypnotist can enable him to control his perception of pain, so that even when he wakens from the trace, the pain is more bearable. The patient can also be taught to hypnotize himself.

PAIN CLINICS

Pain clinics in Britain tend to concentrate on the relief of pain by drugs or injections such as those described in the chapter on back pain. Acupuncture and hypnosis may be included and, less frequently, chiropractic methods.

Pain clinics in the United States, and a few in Britain, employ different methods, based on a combination of methods of treatment, including drugs, TENS and behaviour modification.

As has already been described, people who have been in pain for a long time show typical symptoms. Other people are at first sympathetic, so reinforcing the pain behaviour. Pain clinics of the American type aim at reversing this behaviour pattern. The patient's co-operation is necessary and an agreement is made between patient and clinic. Pain behaviour is ignored, while patients who do not complain and try to be active are praised and encouraged. Analgesics are given in gradually reduced dosage. The family's active co-operation is also necessary. Goals are set and progress monitored.

The use of operant conditioning is similar. Because body and mind are so inextricably linked, the patient may come to associate the pain in his body with the tasks and responsibilities he formerly disliked. A balance must be achieved between the patient's life tasks and his physical condition. The aim of treatment is to enable the patient to live and function with his pain. He enters into a contract to co-operate with the treatment programme and to talk about his pain only to staff, and then only when specifically asked about it. The occupational therapy assessment and treatment plan are similar to that already described, with the addition of the cognitive behavioural approach to pain in which the patient is taught to analyse and identify his own problems and to discover his own ways of dealing with them. Patients have to be made aware of their negative attitudes, and keep a diary of events which trigger tension, then examine with the therapist the sequence of events from this tension being aroused to the way in which the patient's cognition seemed to contribute to the pain. Patients are then taught to interrupt this sequence by re-examining events more rationally and directing their attention elsewhere. The family is involved in the treatment plan, and is able to observe the patient's achievable activity level, so that they can reinforce the treatment.

This last approach is unlikely to be carried out on the orthopaedic ward, but serves as information as to what further treatment is available when conventional methods have failed.

REFERENCES

Brena, S.F. (1978) *Chronic Pain: America's hidden epidemic*, Athenium SMI, New York.

Broome, A. and Jellicoe, H. (1987) *Living with Pain*, British Psychological Society/Methuen, London.

Cailliet, R. (1988) *Low Back Pain Syndrome*, 4th edn, F.A. Davis, Philadelphia.

Chaitow, L. (1985) *Your Complete Stress-Proofing Programme*, Thorsons Publishing Group, Wellingborough.

Hanna, M. (1988) Management of chronic pain, in C.J. Goodwill and M.A. Chamberlain (eds.) *Rehabilitation of the Physically Disabled Adult, Part II*, Croom Helm/Sheridan Medical, London.

Jayson, M.V. (1987) Back Pain: The facts, 2nd edn, Oxford Medical Publications, Oxford.

Melzack, R. and Wall, P.D. (1988) *The Challenge of Pain*, Penguin Books, Harmondsworth.

FURTHER READING

Giles, G.G. and Allen, M.E. (1986) Occupational therapy in the treatment of the patient with chronic pain, *British Journal of Occupational Therapy*, January, 4–8.

Melzack, R. and Dennis, S.G. (1978) Neurophysiological foundations of pain, in R.A. Sternbach (ed.) *The Psychology of Pain*, Raven Press, New York.

Rogers, S.R., Shuer, J. and Herzig, S. (1984) Use of feedback techniques for persons with chronic pain, in P. Cromwell (ed.) *Occupational Therapy and the Patient with Pain*, Haworth Press, New York.

Strong, J. (1987) Chronic pain management: the occupational therapist's role, *British Journal of Occupational Therapy*, August, 262–3.

12

Resettlement

Many orthopaedic patients have problems relating to employment, manifested in taking considerable sick leave through to having ceased work owing to the effects of their disability. The first may need rehabilitation to build up stamina to return to work, the second may need assessment for alternative work and vocational guidance.

The labour market has undergone many changes, with automation leading to fewer manual jobs. With high employment costs, the worker need not be fully fit, but he is required to do the job competently within a specified time limit. Firms who employ more than 20 staff are required by law to employ at least 3% as registered disabled people.

Work improves self-esteem, gives a feeling of usefulness, alleviates depression and facilitates socialization. It implies improved income and enhanced quality of life. It is therefore an essential part of the total rehabilitation and resettlement of the patient.

PRELIMINARY WORK ASSESSMENT

The patient's occupation is stated on his hospital admission form and in her initial assessment the occupational therapist can ask for details of what this work involves. If the patient has had a long period off work, he should be asked if his job is being held open for him. If his previous job is no longer suitable, his firm may consider redeployment. An alternative may be to adapt the job, e.g. by providing suitable equipment or controls or altering the position of work. The patient may be capable of returning to similar work after a period of intensive rehabilitation.

If alternative employment is necessary, local opportunities and training schemes should be explored. A young patient on the threshold of a career may need guidance towards suitable training. Another patient may benefit from sheltered working conditions. For all these situations a basic work assessment is needed. If the individual's potential earning capacity is very low and he would lose benefits, it may be better to channel his energies in another direction.

DETAILED WORK ASSESSMENT

The patient should first be independent in most activities of daily living, including toileting, and independently mobile, with a wheelchair if necessary. He should have reached an advanced stage of rehabilitation, with good balance and co-ordination, and reasonable strength and range of movement commensurate with the type of work he will be seeking. He should also be psychologically ready, with good concentration and motivation.

Ideally the occupational therapist should visit the patient's place of work to obtain an accurate picture of the working conditions and to see precisely what the work entails. Is the work indoor or outdoor, clean or dirty, noisy or quiet, alone or with others? Is there machinery? Is there a production line in which the workers are interdependent, resulting in pressure to keep up the pace? Is the work stimulating and varied, or is it repetitive and potentially boring? Any particular skills required for the job should be noted, including the position in the work hierarchy, communication skills, relationships with employer and fellow employees and ability to make decisions or use initiative.

The patient's physical capacity to walk about, stand for any length of time, sit in comfort, lift or carry heavy or awkward objects, bend down, stretch up, climb ladders, operate machinery or drive must be assessed as appropriate. Balance, co-ordination, manual dexterity and adequate sensation in the hand are required in varying degrees for most jobs. Speed of work is an important factor. Strong grasp of the type appropriate to the work is necessary, e.g. power grip for wielding a hammer, tripod grip for holding a pen, etc. Clumsiness, tremor or lack of sensation may be a hazard.

If alternative employment is required, it is necessary to carry out a work assessment to enable the patient to be matched with a job vacancy. This differs somewhat from the previous procedure. The work in which the patient was previously engaged is relevant but various areas of work may be tested, including manual, clerical and technical. Contracted-out work or processes carried out in various hospital departments may be used for this purpose, and the results of any productive work must be examined for quality. Literacy, numeracy and learning capacity are assessed. The patient is instructed by demonstration, and by verbal and written means, to discover his best learning method. Psychological assessment includes observation of his interactions with his fellow 'workers' and relationship with his supervisor, and his dependence on others. His attitude towards work is assessed, including the interest and motivation he displays, his ability to make decisions, concentrate, show initiative, manage time effectively and cope with pressure. His appearance is noted, attendance record and punctuality monitored, and an opinion formed as to his reliability and honesty. The assessment is documented under the following broad headings:

- name, address, date of birth and diagnosis;
- former employment and/or educational attainments;
- physical assessment;
- psychological assessment;
- preferred method of learning;
- type of work thought to be most suited to the patient.

REHABILITATION TOWARDS RETURN TO WORK

If the occupational therapy department has the facilities to simulate the patient's workplace, rehabilitation may be carried out there. The patient is required to arrive at the department independently and on time, appropriately attired. He should bring his packed lunch or buy his lunch as he would at the works canteen. The speed at which he works and the hours he puts in should gradually approximate to his normal work, so that he builds up stamina for a full working day. Any difficulties should be discussed with the employer, with a view to solving them possibly by the provision of adapted tools, equipment or improved access.

The link between occupational therapy work assessment and the Employment Rehabilitation Centre

There is a nationwide network of Employment Rehabilitation Centres (ERCs). Ideally the patient should progress routinely from the medical scene in hospital to the employment rehabilitation scene at the ERC. Relatively few occupational therapy departments have the staff or the facilities to operate a dynamic work rehabilitation programme. Where these facilities are needed, the therapist may recommend referral to the ERC as being in the patient's best interests. Because medical staff have contact with occupational therapists, it is to them that patients are referred for work assessment. However, if the patient is referred to the Disablement Resettlement Officer (DRO) based at the Job Centre, he is likely to be referred on to the ERC for assessment.

The average length of attendance at the ERC is approximately six weeks. Because it is equipped like a factory and run on similar lines, the setting is more realistic. The work available includes electrical work, electronics, assembly work, engineering, joinery, gardening, commercial and business work. Physical exercise sessions are incorporated and clients are trained in seeking work and interview techniques. Note that the patient has now become the client, a subtle difference which gives a psychological boost. His progress is regularly reviewed by a team composed of the ERC manager, the DRO, a medical officer, a social worker and a psychologist.

The assessment of each client is broken down into six component parts, which are necessary for every client and every type of work, although the relative importance of each part varies from one job to another. These components include assessment of:

- the medical condition;
- the physical capacity at the time, and the projected potential after rehabilitation;
- the psychological state, including adjustment to the physical disability;
- intelligence, literacy and numeracy;
- social skills;
- ability in practical skills.

While attending the ERC clients are paid a maintenance allowance.

The Disablement Resettlement Officer

The DRO is responsible for placing disabled people in employment. He advises on training schemes, vocational guidance, suitable job vacancies and alternative employment. He may require confidential reports from the doctor and from the occupational therapist regarding work assessment.

He may suggest that his client registers as a disabled person on the register maintained by the Department of Employment. Patients have to be substantially disabled for at least a year to be eligible for this register. Being registered may facilitate the finding of a suitable job, especially in reserved occupations such as passenger lift attendants and car park attendants, and in Sheltered Placement Schemes (SPS). SPS are sponsored by Remploy, many local authorities and voluntary bodies and offer sheltered work in factory conditions in a wide variety of jobs, usually under contract from local firms. Workers are paid a living wage and are expected to work a standard working week, although their pace is slower than that required in the open market. The sponsor is the employer and their costs are offset by the host firm's contribution in wages, plus a contribution from the Department of Employment.

Other help available through the DRO includes:

- The Job Introduction Scheme: an allowance of £45 per week (1992) to be paid to an employer for a six week trial period if he takes on a disabled person about whose ability he is doubtful.
- If work is considered to be part of the rehabilitation process for a disabled person recommended by a doctor and approved by the Department of Health, earnings of £40.50 per week (1992) are allowed without having to surrender Invalidity Benefit.
- Contact for application for training at any of the five residential training colleges for disabled people, offering courses of approximately six months duration, covering clerical work, telephonist and reception work,

gardening, electronics, woodwork, etc. The colleges are distributed across England, at Banstead Place, Surrey (school leavers); Finchale Training College, Durham; Portland Training College, Mansfield; Queen Elizabeth Training College, Leatherhead; and St. Loyes College, Exeter.

- A grant for a person on the disabled persons register who incurs extra travel costs to work because of his disability.
- Schemes to provide special tools or equipment to enable a disabled person to work.

The Disablement Advisory Service

The Disablement Advisory Service (DAS) links up with the services of the DRO. Both are contactable at the local Job Centre, and the DAS offers:

- provision of funds for modified machinery or adaptations at the workplace, e.g. ramps, lifts, adapted toilets, etc., for a specific disabled person. The maximum grant is £6000 (1992);
- a data bank of information available to employers and occupational therapists to enable disabled people to overcome problems encountered at work;
- advice and practical help to employers on how to use the skills of disabled employees to the full, and gives ongoing support;
- advice and assistance in setting up schemes for home-based work in information technology.

Royal Society for Disability and Rehabilitation (RADAR)

This organization provides information regarding employment-related difficulties. Their Mobility Officer will provide details on local schemes to enable disabled people to get to and from work. The organizer of the Rehabilitation Engineering Movement Advisory Panel (REMAP) supplies addresses of local panels who design and make up one-off adaptations or tools to overcome a specific problem at work. Labour is free but a charge may be made for materials. The Housing/Access Officer of RADAR and the Centre for Accessible Environment advise on adaptations to premises to accommodate a disabled worker (addresses in appendix).

COMPENSATION

A patient with a compensation case pending may consciously or unconsciously hold back on progress. Unfortunately, compensation cases often take years to reach a settlement. Meanwhile the solicitor sometimes advises the patient to limit his activities in order to obtain more in damages. This delays recovery.

The situation is further aggravated if the solicitor does not want the patient to return to work until after the claim is settled. The longer he remains off sick, the more difficult it is to settle back into work. Because of loss of earnings as a result of an injury, the patient is naturally eager to gain as much in compensation as possible.

In the case of a compensation case pending, occupational therapy progress must be well documented so that an accurate report can be compiled if requested by the solicitor.

Not every patient with a compensation case pending exhibits 'compensation neurosis', but if satisfactory progress is not being made, this may well be worth considering.

SOCIAL RESETTLEMENT

Resettlement at home has been implicit in each chapter, and we have now considered resettlement at work. An essential part of the latter is the patient's ability to travel to and from work. Transport is also the key to resettlement into the community. Most patients on discharge home are mobile about the house, using a walking aid if necessary, but out-of-doors mobility may be very limited. A wheelchair or car adaptations may be necessary.

Wheelchairs

Wheelchair assessment for patients who have rheumatoid arthritis and who have had lower limb amputation has been covered in the relevant chapters. Others may need a wheelchair in the short term, e.g. while they are non-weightbearing or while they are immobilized in long leg cylinder plasters. A wheelchair may be obtainable for short-term loan from the District Wheelchair Service, Social Services or from a voluntary body such as the British Red Cross Society. Fittings such as elevating legrests may not be readily available, and it may expedite provision if the resources of the heavy workshop or the hospital works department are tapped, to make up L-shaped padded boards. These are made comfortable by placing one cushion on the seat part. A wheelchair with an elevating leg-rest is awkward to manoeuvre in tight corners, knocking into people and objects, but fortunately they are rarely needed for a long period.

Patients who need wheelchairs for long-term use require a more detailed assessment, with re-assessment at regular intervals to ensure that their needs are being met. Such patients are those with neurological disorders, paraplegia, tetraplegia, etc. who may need orthopaedic surgery for release of contractures, spinal surgery, etc. For these patients, the following points should be considered when choosing a suitable model:

- Is the wheelchair for regular or occasional use?
- Is it to be used indoors or out?
- If for indoors, are doors wide enough, and is there adequate turning space?
- Which is the most appropriate model: self-propelled, attendant pushed or electric?
- Is it to be used on rough or hilly terrain?
- What does the patient intend to do while in the wheelchair: cook, deskwork, go shopping, gardening, etc.?
- Is a folding model needed, for carrying in a car boot? (An L by the model number in the NHS list indicates lightweight.)
- Are any special features necessary: rear wheels set back, reclining back rest, etc.?
- Are any extra features necessary: tray, desk armrests, safety strap, etc.?
- Is a pressure cushion needed?

The patient's height and weight are recorded on the referral form, with the diagnosis and any physical or mental problems which might affect his ability to control the wheelchair. An electrically powered model may be more appropriate for the patient with progressive disease. The needs and ability of an attendant are important; he may not be fit enough to push the laden wheelchair up a slope or lift it into a car boot. Most NHS wheelchairs have detachable armrests and adjustable foot-rests which swing outwards to facilitate getting in and out. Backrest angles vary, and folding backrests are much less supportive, although a bracing device is available. Elevating legrests and supportive seating are needed on models with a fully reclining backrest.

Patients with limited shoulder extension may be unable to reach rear propelling wheels on standard models, but the Bencraft six wheeler has the propelling wheels directly beneath the shoulder joints. Front propelling wheels pose problems as the legrests do not swing outwards, although the footrests flip upward to allow access from the front of the wheelchair. If the patient has to do a sideways transfer, the large front wheels are an obstacle, especially in models with larger wheels. Larger castors are more stable and cope better with rough ground and kerbs. Brake levers must be well within the patient's reach, with extended levers if the grip is weak to make them easier to operate. Solid tyres may be preferred on indoor wheelchairs, but pneumatic tyres absorb shock on an outdoor model. If any tyres become worn or are not maintained at the correct pressure, the brakes will not be effective.

Mobile arm support attachments are available for patients with very weak upper limbs, as in muscular dystrophy, tetraplegia or severe rheumatoid arthritis. One-arm drive wheelchairs are rarely needed for orthopaedic patients. The wheelchairs supplied through the District Wheelchair Service are adequate for the needs of most patients. If the patient is wheelchair bound, he is supplied with an indoor and an outdoor model, the latter being heavier and more robust. If he lives on two levels with a connecting stairlift, he is allowed a further wheelchair for use upstairs. He will have two pairs of armrests if appropriate, for domestic use and for office work. He is supplied with a manual of instructions for use and maintenance to ensure safety, with details of the local contact for repair, which is free. It is essential that the patient quotes his reference number when requesting repair. He can obtain this number by contacting the District Wheelchair Service.

Although the range of statutory chairs has been extended, a much wider range is available commercially. The younger patient confined to a wheelchair usually obtains a lightweight model which is very manoeuvrable, but this is not usually supplied by the District Wheelchair Service.

A patient who is unable to raise himself by his arms to relieve the pressure on his bottom needs anti-pressure cushioning, to which he is entitled along with the wheelchair and for which he is individually assessed. Available cushions include sculpted foam, water and foam, gel, air cell and silicone types. The patient with scoliosis, if not completely corrected by surgery, will also need lateral support in the form of foam fit systems or swing-away thoracic supports.

If the wheelchair is to be used long-term, ramps are necessary wherever access is required. In the short-term, temporary portable ramps can be supplied quickly at low cost. The gradient of the ramp should be no more than 1 in 12, the surface must be non-skid and the side edges raised.

A person confined to a wheelchair is at a disadvantage in company. People carrying on a conversation while standing will be talking over his head. A Mangar booster will enable the permanently chairbound person to raise himself to talk to standing colleagues face-to-face.

Mobility allowance

This is a non-contributory benefit payable to an individual who is unable, or virtually unable, to walk for at least 12 months. It is payable whether the claimant works or not, provided he satisfies the medical, residential and age conditions. A doctor appointed by the Department of Health assesses the patient's mobility, using whatever walking aid is appropriate. If the walking ability is likely to improve a short-term award is made, lasting for a minimum of a year. If the walking disability is permanent, the allowance may be made up to the age of 80 years, providing the application was made before the age of 65 years. Payment of Mobility Allowance is not affected by periods in hospital or residential care, but is affected by certain other criteria. For full details, see DHSS Leaflet HB5 (DHSS, 1990).

Persons receiving Mobility Allowance may be entitled to certain other benefits. Among these are:

- exemption from Road Tax;
- inclusion in the Orange Badge Scheme;
- entitlement to drive at the age of 16 years;
- exemption form vat when buying motability cars and car adaptations;
- medical exemption from wearing a seat belt;
- british railcard for disabled people;
- severe disablement allowance if of working age but unable to work;
- disability premium in calculating Income Support and Housing Benefit.

The Motability scheme was set up to enable people with Mobility Allowance to obtain a car or electric wheelchair at a reduced price. Cars may be bought on hire purchase or hired, and electric wheelchairs may be acquired on hire purchase. The person receiving Mobility Allowance agrees to Social Security paying all or part of the allowance to Motability Finance Ltd for the duration of the lease or hire agreement. The Mobility Allowance award must be for at least the period of the lease or hire agreement. Any extra cost must be paid in a lump sum at the outset, and this includes the cost of any adaptations to the car (full details in DHSS Leaflet HB 5).

The Orange Badge Scheme enables appreciably disabled people to park in restricted areas, to facilitate access to shops, banks, places of entertainment, etc. The badge must be displayed on the windscreen. It entitles the holder to park for up to two hours on double yellow lines, free parking at parking meters and parking without a time limit in limited waiting areas. The holder must not park where he causes obstruction or a hazard. The badge is obtained through the Social Services department.

The Motability facility and Orange Badge Scheme may be used by the carer on behalf of the disabled person if he is unable to drive himself.

The disabled driver

The patient with limited mobility may be very dependent on his car to go to work, the shops, or for social contact. It may be impossible for him to manage public transport. The doctor in charge of the case has to judge whether the individual is competent to drive, and the orthopaedic patient with no neurological dysfunction or psychiatric problem is usually deemed fit. Most patients merely require a car with automatic transmission and possibly power-assisted steering. The occupational therapist may have to carry out a basic assessment in the patient's own car. This will include the patient's ability to get in and out of the car, suitability of the driving seat, manipulation of the controls and pinpointing what adaptations are necessary. This is adequate for most patients but if the condition is progressive or he has had an amputation, a specialist assessment may be needed. The Mobility Centre at Banstead Place or the

Mobility Advice and Vehicle Information Service (MAVIS) set up by the Department of Transport may be of assistance (addresses in appendix).

The range of movement required for driving is not great. More than 65° of flexion deformity at elbow or knee causes problems. Limitation of hip flexion can usually be accommodated by inclining the backrest of the driving seat slightly. Limited shoulder movement is of little consequence. Weak grip or loss of an arm may be overcome by fitting a steering wheel knob.

Results of assessments of various adaptations for cars have been recorded in the DHSS Disability Equipment Assessment Programme. Their reports cover the assessment of backrests, replacement car seats, supplementary mirrors (necessary where there are cervical problems), handbrake adaptations and steering wheel knobs. The Scoliosis Association publish an information sheet on 'Scoliosis and car seats'.

Car conversions may be carried out by the main car manufacturers or by specialist companies. Types of conversions include alteration of the accelerator pedal from right to left side, conversion to hand controls, or power steering, joystick steering, switch extensions, handbrake release and conversions for passengers. Tail lifts can be fitted to the rear of some vehicles. A swivel seat can be fitted to either front seat, to enable it to be swung round by 90° to enable easier entrance and exit. For the severely disabled, hoists and lifts are available. Automatic garage doors are useful although car ports may be preferable. The disabled driver may require help at a self-service petrol station, or if he is in trouble on the motorway. Various 'Help' signals are on the market, and certain motoring organizations offer specific help to the disabled motorist.

A person who develops a disability which may affect his driving ability must inform the Driving and Vehicle Licensing Centre (DVLC) at Swansea. The DVLC Medical Advisory Branch may then require a medical examination and report. The insurance company must also be informed of any disability which may affect driving capability.

Because of limitations on the therapist's time, a file or leaflet containing relevant information on driving should be made available to the patient to give him encouragement in picking up the threads of his life again.

Leisure activities

Leisure activity fulfils certain needs. It enables a person to relax, meet and perhaps compete with others with like interests, gives opportunities for self-development, leadership and creativity, and may be used as an alternative to employment. It provides opportunities for achievement and the means of retaining or regaining self-esteem.

Patients should be encouraged to resume their former interests if possible, and if necessary the means of adapting these activities to the present situation should be explored. If the patient is unable to resume previous interests, he needs information in order to experiment with new ones. He needs to be able to contribute to any group he joins and not simply be on the receiving end. The aim is to integrate into community activities if possible, and Physically Handicapped and Able-Bodied (PHAB) clubs are useful.

The choice of activity must be within the patient's capabilities. It requires courage to attempt something new and he needs the support of family and friends. Research into what is available must take into account travel to the venue and its accessibility to the person concerned. Equipment or tools can be adapted if necessary, either by a little ingenuity or by REMAP.

Membership of specific societies will provide information on necessary equipment, and the *Directory of Grant-Making Trusts* (Charities Aid Foundation, 1991) provides details of charities who will consider making a contribution towards the cost of such equipment. This directory is usually available in the reference section of public libraries.

Frequently contact sports are contra-indicated for orthopaedic patients, but other sporting activities may be suggested. Swimming is excellent exercise and many public baths set aside a time when the baths are open solely for disabled people and their families for their greater comfort. Horse riding, sailing, camping and the Disabled Olympics are possibilities, and people with disarticulation of the hip have learned to ski. Spectator sports lead to social integration.

Gardening is within the reach of any disabled person, using adapted tools and a suitably planned garden. Various specialist societies cater for all tastes, e.g. alpines, cacti, fuchsias, etc. For specific help Horticultural Therapy may be approached, and Gardens for the Disabled Trust make grants to adapt garden layouts and purchase special tools. There are several demonstration gardens nationwide and gardening is frequently used in sheltered employment. Merely tending his own front garden or window box, a disabled person will meet passers-by and thereby become involved with the local community.

While some disabled people are unable to go out to pursue their interests or prefer to use their computer or knitting machine at home, others wish to engage in cultural activities, go to concerts or the theatre, visit libraries, museums and art galleries. This should be encouraged, plus active participation in the fields of music, art and drama. The arts bring great pleasure to those who practise them and to those who observe. People can discover hidden talents and a creative outlet, can share ideas and experiences, and develop physical and perceptual skills. There are theatre companies who employ disabled actors, who are exploring new areas of artistic experience for both actors and audiences. Access to the relevant public buildings and the provision of toilet facilities is steadily improving.

Disabled people and their families need holidays either together or separately: the choice should be theirs. Most holiday brochures state whether they have facilities for people with disabilities, and lists of special accommodation are published by organizations such as RADAR. Arthritis Care runs several holiday hotels. Transport advice is available from RADAR and from Holiday Care Service; the latter also provide experienced volunteers to help disabled people on holiday and may help with funding. More organized holidays can be booked via Across, which caters for holidays abroad. The occupational therapy department should make this type of information available to patients, as many of them look forward to a holiday when they are better. Having information to hand enables them to make positive plans and may help with goal setting. Once a holiday has been undertaken, social resettlement is well under way.

QUALITY OF LIFE

While retraining in the activities of daily living and provision of tools and adaptations make up the largest part of the resettlement programme, it is important that the further aspects of resettlement discussed in this chapter are addressed. These contribute to quality of life, which encompasses all features of the person's integration into the community, including any means of minimizing his disability. Employment, social and leisure activities contribute to this enrichment of life.

Quality of life may be judged by four criteria (Blunden, 1988). These are physical, cognitive, material and social well-being. While the patients we have been considering may be somewhat lacking in physical well-being, the remaining three areas are open to them. Cognitive well-being can be summed up as being content with one's lot, and material well-being as having an adequate income, a home and some means of transport. Social well-being entails being known, respected and valued on one's own merits, with choice in as many areas as possible, and competence in mobility and communication skills. The social dimension of quality of life tends to be overlooked in the provision of services for people with disabilities. The Attenborough Report on Arts and Disabled People (Carnegie UK Trust, 1985) does not accept that the arts are no more than the 'icing on the cake'. The occupational therapist is well placed to make any relevant information available and point her patient towards full social resettlement.

REFERENCES

Blunden, R. (1988) Quality of life in persons with disabilities: issues in the development of services, in R.I. Brown (ed.) *Quality of Life for Handicapped People*, Croom Helm, London.

Carnegie UK Trust (1985) *The Attenborough Report: Arts and disabled people*, Bedford Square Press/NCVO, London.

Charities Aid Foundation (1991) *Directory of Grant-Making Trusts*, CAF, Tonbridge.

Department of Health and Social Security (1984–1986) *Disability Equipment Assessment Programme Booklets*, DHSS Publications Unit, Heywood, Lancs.

Department of Health and Social Security (1990) *A Guide to Non-Contributory Benefits for Disabled People*, Leaflet HB5, DHSS Publications Unit, Heywood, Lancs.

FURTHER READING

Clarke, A., Allard, L. and Braybrooks, B. (1987) *Rehabilitation in Rheumatology: The team approach*, Martin Dunitz, London.

Disabled Living Foundation (1988) *Information Service Handbook*, Sections 6 and 8, Disabled Living Foundation, London.

Employment Service Leaflets (1990) Available from local Employment Service offices, address in Telephone Directory.

Goodwill, J. (1988) Car driving for the disabled, in C.J. Goodwill and M.A. Chamberlain (eds.) *Rehabilitation of the Physically Disabled Adult*, Croom Helm/Sheridan Medical, London.

Kennedy, M. (1986) Able to work? *British Journal of Occupational Therapy*, November, 354–6.

Nichols, P.J.R. *et al.* (1980) *Rehabilitation Medicine: The management of physical disabilities*, 2nd edn, Butterworths, London.

Occupational Therapists' Reference Book (1990) Parke Sutton Ltd/British Association of Occupational Therapists, Norwich.

Turner, A. (ed.) (1981) *The Practice of Occupational Therapy: An introduction to the treatment of physical dysfunction*, Churchill Livingstone, Edinburgh.

Western, P. (1987) Leisure pursuits, in E. Bumphrey (ed.) *Occupational Therapy in the Community*, Woodhead-Faulkner, Cambridge.

Appendix

ACROSS TRUST

Bridge House, 70/72 Bridge Road,
East Molesey, Surrey KT8 9HF
081-783-1355

ARTHRITIS CARE

5 Grosvenor Crescent, London
SW 1X 7ER
071-235-0902

ARTHRITIS AND RHEUMATISM COUNCIL

Copeman House, St. Mary's Court,
St. Mary's Gate,
Chesterfield S41 7TD
0246-558033

BACUP (BRITISH ASSOCIATION OF CANCER UNITED PATIENTS)

121/123 Charterhouse Street, London EC1 M 6AA
071-608-1661
(Also FREEPHONE for calls outside London: 0800-181199)

BANSTEAD MOBILITY CENTRE

Damson Way, Orchard Hill,
Queen Mary's Avenue, Carshalton, Surrey S5 4 NR
081-7701151

BRITISH AMPUTEE SPORTS ASSOCIATION

(Contact) Mr John Fisher, 17 Douglas Road,
Harpenden, Herts AL5 2EN
0582-460105

BRITISH SPORTS ASSOCIATION FOR THE DISABLED

34 Osnaburgh Street, London NW1 3ND
071-383-7277

BRITISH RED CROSS SOCIETY

9 Grosvenor Crescent, London
SW 1X 7EJ
071-235-5454

CAMPING FOR THE DISABLED

20 Burton Close, Dawley, Telford,
Shropshire TF 4 2 BX
0743-761889 (Daytime)
0952-507653 (Evenings)

CANCER RELIEF MACMILLAN FUND

15/19 Britten Street,
London SW 3 3 TZ
071-351-7811

CANCERLINK

17 Britannia Street, London
WC 1X 9JN
071-833-2451

CENTRE FOR ACCESSIBLE ENVIRONMENT

35 Great Smith Street,
London SW1P 3BJ
071-222-7980

COMPUTABILITY-CENTRE

c/o Mr Tom Mangan,
P O Box 94,
Warwick CV34 5WS
0926-312847

DHSS AIDS ASSESSMENT PROGRAMME

DHSS Store
Health Publications Unit,
No. 2. Site,
Manchester Road,
Heywood, Lancs OL10 2PZ
0706-366287

DISABLED DRIVERS' ASSOCIATION

Ashwellthorpe Hall,
Ashwellthorpe, Norwich, Norfolk
NR16 1EX
050841-449

DISABLED LIVING FOUNDATION

Clothing and Footwear Advisory Service,
380/384 Harrow Road,
London W9 2HU
071-289-6111

DISABLED PHOTOGRAPHERS' SOCIETY

PO Box 130, Richmond,
Surrey TW10 6XQ

EQUIPMENT FOR DISABLED PEOPLE

Publications from:
Mary Marlborough Lodge,
Nuffield Orthopaedic Centre,
Headington, Oxford OX3 7LD
0865-750103

GARDENING FOR THE DISABLED TRUST

Julia Sebline, Secretary,
Hayes Farm House, Hayes Lane,
Peasmarsh, Nr.Rye, East Sussex TN31 6XR

HOLIDAY CARE SERVICE

2 Old Bank Chambers, Station Road, Horley
Surrey RH6 9 HW
0293-774535

HOMECRAFT SUPPLIES LTD.

Siding Road,
Low Moor Estate,
Kirby-in-Ashfield,
Nottingham NG17 7JZ
0623-754047
Supply Droopsnoot and Balans type chairs

HORTICULTURAL THERAPY

Goulds Ground, Vallis Way, Frome,
Somerset BA11 3DW
0373-464782

MAUBRI FASHIONS

Unit 13 B, Springfield Industrial Estate,
Farsley, Leeds LS28 5 LY
0532-553274

MAVIS (MOBILITY ADVICE AND VEHICLE INFORMATION SERVICE)

Department of Transport,
Transport and Road Research Laboratory,
Crowthorne, Berks RG11 6AU
0344-770456

NATIONAL ANKYLOSING SPONDYLITIS SOCIETY

5 Grosvenor Crescent, London SW1X 7ER
071-235-9585

NALD (NATIONAL ASSOCIATION FOR LIMBLESS DISABLED)

31 The Mall, Ealing, London W5 2PX

081-579-1758/9

NATIONAL BACK PAIN ASSOCIATION

31/33 Park Road, Teddington, Middx

TW 11 OAB

081-977-5474

PHAB (PHYSICALLY HANDICAPPED AND ABLE BODIED)

National Office, 12/14 London Rd, Croydon

CR0 2TA

081-667-9443

PILGRIM'S PRESS

Caxton House, Ongar,

Essex CM5 9RB

0277-364060

PUTNAMS

Eastern Wood Road,

Langage,

Plympton,

Devon PL7 5ET

0752-345678

Supply Putnam Wedge

RADAR (ROYAL ASSOCIATION FOR DISABILITY AND REHABILITATION)
REMAP (REHABILITATION ENGINEERING MOVEMENT ADVISORY PANELS)

BOTH THE ABOVE AT:

25 Mortimer Street,

London W1N 8 AB

071-637-5400

REMPLOY LTD

415 Edgware Road, Cricklewood,
London NW2 6 LR
081-452-8020

RIDING FOR THE DISABLED ASSOCIATION

Avenue R, National Agricultural Centre,
Kenilworth, Warwicks CV8 2LY
0203-696510

SCOLIOSIS ASSOCIATION (UK)

2 Ivebury Court,
325 Latimer Road,
London W10 6RA
081-964-5343

SPOD (SEXUAL AND PERSONAL RELATIONSHIPS OF THE DISABLED)

286 Campden Road, London N7 OBJ
071-607-8851

A.J. WAY & CO. LTD

Unit 2,
Sunters End,
Hillbottom Road,
Sands Industrial Estate,
High Wycombe,
Bucks HP12 4HZ
0494-471821
Supply Droopsnoot chair

WIDER HORIZONS

(an organization for promoting wider interests among handicapped people)
Hon. Administrator/Treasurer,
Mr A.B. Fletcher, Westbrook,
Back Lane, Malvern, Worcs WR14 2HJ

INDEX